> ## "America's leading source of self-help legal information." ★★★★
> —YAHOO!

LEGAL INFORMATION ONLINE ANYTIME

24 hours a day

www.nolo.com

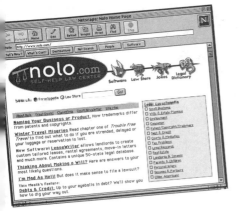

AT THE NOLO.COM SELF-HELP LAW CENTER, YOU'LL FIND

- Nolo's comprehensive Legal Encyclopedia filled with plain-English information on a variety of legal topics
- Nolo's Law Dictionary—legal terms <u>without</u> the legalese
- Auntie Nolo—if you've got questions, Auntie's got answers
- The Law Store—over 250 self-help legal products including: Downloadable Software, Books, Form Kits and eGuides
- Legal and product updates
- Frequently Asked Questions
- NoloBriefs, our free monthly email newsletter
- Legal Research Center, for access to state and federal statutes
- Our ever-popular lawyer jokes

Quality LAW BOOKS & SOFTWARE FOR EVERYONE

Nolo's user-friendly products are consistently first-rate. Here's why:

- A dozen in-house legal editors, working with highly skilled authors, ensure that our products are accurate, up-to-date and easy to use
- We continually update every book and software program to keep up with changes in the law
- Our commitment to a more democratic legal system informs all of our work
- We appreciate & listen to your feedback. Please fill out and return the card at the back of this book.

OUR "NO-HASSLE" GUARANTEE

Return anything you buy directly from Nolo for any reason and we'll cheerfully refund your purchase price. No ifs, ands or buts.

An Important Message to Our Readers

This product provides information and general advice about the law. But laws and procedures change frequently, and they can be interpreted differently by different people. For specific advice geared to your specific situation, consult an expert. No book, software or other published material is a substitute for personalized advice from a knowledgeable lawyer licensed to practice law in your state.

3rd Edition

Beat the Nursing Home Trap:

A Consumer's Guide to Assisted Living and Long-Term Care

by Joseph Matthews

Keeping Up-to-Date

To keep its books up to date, Nolo issues new printings and new editions periodically. New printings reflect minor legal changes and technical corrections. New editions contain major legal changes, major text additions or major reorganizations. To find out if a later printing or edition of any Nolo book is available, call Nolo at 510-549-1976 or check our website at www.nolo.com.

To stay current, follow the "Update" service at our website: www.nolo.com. In another effort to help you use Nolo's latest materials, we offer a 35% discount off the purchase of the new edition of your Nolo book when you turn in the cover of an earlier edition. (See the "Special Upgrade Offer" in the back of the book.)

This book was last revised in: OCTOBER 1999.

THIRD EDITION	October 1999
EDITOR	Barbara Kate Repa
BOOK DESIGN	Jackie Mancuso
COVER DESIGN	Toni Ihara
ILLUSTRATIONS	IMSI (in San Rafael); The Learning Company ("©1996 The Learning Company Inc. and its licensors.")
INDEX	Nancy Mulvany
PRINTING	Bertelsmann Industry Services, Inc.

Matthews, Joseph L.
    Beat the nursing home trap : a consumer's guide to choosing & financing long-term care / by Joseph Matthews. -- 3rd ed.
    p. cm.
  Includes index.
  ISBN 0-87337-515-7
  1. Aged—Long term care--Evaluation. 2. Long-term care of the sick--Evaluation. 3. Aged--Long-term care--Finance. 4. Long-term care of the sick--Finance. 5. Consumer education. I. Title.
RA644.5 .M38 1999
362.1'6--dc21   98-51467
                                                          CIP

Acknowledgments

Many thanks go to Ralph Warner, who saw immediately the value of a book such as this and who gave the project its birth.

Special thanks go to Peter Yedidia, President of Geriatric Health Systems of San Francisco, who gave generously of his time and vast professional experience in matters of health care programs for the elderly. His corrective commentaries greatly strengthened the manuscript.

Special thanks also to Diane Arnold-Driver, Coordinator of the Center on Aging at the University of California, Berkeley. She shared readily her great expertise in geriatric care matters and tactfully made a number of suggestions which redounded to the significant benefit of the text.

Thank you also to Lora Connolly and Sandra Pierce-Miller of the California Department of Health Services who took the time to clarify a number of matters pertaining to state partnership long-term care insurance programs.

And many thanks to Stan Jacobsen, whose thorough research has not only helped keep this book up-to-date, but has also provided readers with valuable new information.

A final and most exuberant thanks goes to my editor, Barbara Kate Repa, whose perspicacity and skill are matched only by her patience and good humor. She needed all of them with me. The quality of this book is in large measure due to her talents.

Contents

1
Making Decisions About Long-Term Care

2

At-Home Care

3

Organized Senior Residences

4

Nursing Facilities

5

Medicare and Veterans' Benefits

6

Medicaid Coverage for Long-Term Care

7

Medicaid and Asset Protection

8.

Protecting Choices About Medical Care and Finances

9

Estate Planning: Controlling Your Money and Property

10

Long-Term Care Insurance

Appendix

Resource Directory

Making Decisions About Long-Term Care

A truth most everyone must face is that you or a family member may someday need some kind of expensive long-term care. Most older people, even if they remain basically healthy, develop physical or mental frailties or impairments which at some point prevent them from living completely independent lives.

More than five million older people in the United States receive some form of daily care at home, provided by someone from outside the family. Millions more receive regular, if not daily, care. And still more millions receive at-home care entirely from family members who will not be able to continue that care indefinitely. In addition to that are nearly two million people over age 65 living full-time in some type of nursing facility or other residential care facility, at a cost of between $20,000 and $100,000 per year. Of people over 65 in nursing facilities, about 25% will live there for more than a year; about 10% more than three years.

Medicare, often thought to "cover" medical care for everyone over 65, in fact pays for only about two percent of all nursing facility costs and only a fraction of all home care costs. Medicaid, the federal government program which pays medical costs for the financially needy, pays for about half of all nursing facility costs, but it requires you to spend most of your personal assets before you can become eligible for coverage. And while Medicaid pays for residence in a few assisted living, shelter care or residential care facilities, most of this cost must be paid with private funds.

These statistics convey an urgent, unsettling message. This book's response to that message is to help you prepare for the likelihood of long-term care by presenting the alternatives you need to consider. The more physically, emotionally and financially prepared you are, and the more in control of your own life, the better off you and your family will be.

A. What Is Long-Term Care?

As used in this book, "long-term care" means regular assistance with medical care (nursing, medicating, physical therapy) or personal needs (eating, dressing, bathing, moving around) provided by someone outside an older person's family. There are many varieties of long-term care—ranging from part-time home care, to adult daycare, to independent living and assisted living residential communities, to nursing facilities. Some long-term care is temporary—for example, recovering from a broken hip or a stroke. Often, though, once begun it lasts for the remainder of an older person's life.

B. Complex Questions of Long-Term Care

An older person's debilitating condition may be only partial—such as failing hearing or eyesight, memory loss, weakness in arms or legs. Or it may be extreme—the effects of a major stroke or heart ailment, overall frailty, the later stages of Alzheimer's disease. Whatever the specific nature of the loss, the need for either temporary or permanent care raises a number of difficult questions:

- What kind of care is needed?
- Who will provide it?
- Where will it be provided?
- How much will it cost?
- Who will pay for it?

Attempting to answer these questions involves negotiating a number of minefields: finding the right level and amount of care, avoiding unnecessary institutionalization, understanding complicated Medicare and Medicaid rules, considering private long-term care insurance—and importantly, paying for the high cost of care without losing every cent you have.

And if the elder is unable to arrange for the care needed, or is not fully aware of the need for care, the burden of providing care may fall heavily on other family members. Spouses and grown children often must take on major if not total responsibility for organizing and paying for long-term care. This book, then, is a guide not just for the elder who needs long-term care, but for all those who will participate in organizing, providing and paying for that care. The book explains financial planning for long-term care: what Medicare and Medicaid pay, whether to buy long-term care insurance, how some of an elder's assets might be protected from long-term care costs. The book emphasizes the need to explore the many care alternatives to nursing homes and guides you in choosing home care, a residential care facility or a nursing facility if that becomes necessary.

And the book explains legal devices and documents that can help protect an elder's dignity and ensure that wishes for medical procedures and property management are followed if he or she can no longer make decisions alone.

1. How This Book Guides You and Your Family

Many people, at many different stages in the process of deciding about how and where to get long-term care, will find guidance in this book.

■ *If your parent, grandparent or other older relative is no longer able to live a fully independent life, and you face questions of where additional care will come from, where your elder relative will live to receive that care, who will pay for it and how:*

Of particular help to you may be the explanation in Section G of this chapter of how a geriatric care manager can organize a program of care for your relative, especially if the elder lives in a different city or state from you. In addition, Chapters 3 and 4 discuss in detail how to choose the right kind and level of elder housing or nursing facility for your relative, and how to make sure the facility will provide a comfortable and humane residential setting.

Chapters 5 through 7 explain how much you can expect Medicare, Medicaid and other government programs to pay for long-term care, and how much of your relative's assets and income he or she will be able to retain or transfer to others. Throughout the book you will also find referrals to agencies and organizations that can provide detailed information and assistance about specific long-term care needs; this information is also collected in a Resource Directory in the Appendix of the book.

■ *If you or a family member are over fifty and want to begin planning to protect your home and other assets from the potential financial disaster of future long-term care:*

In addition to the chapters on Medicare and Medicaid financing, you will find several other chapters particularly valuable. Chapter 7 discusses ways it may be possible to make long-range plans to protect some of your assets from future long-term care costs. Chapter 8 explores ways to preserve your dignity and to retain the most control over your life and property when you are no longer physically or mentally able to handle all your own affairs. Chapter 9 gives an overview of estate planning techniques that can be used to protect an elder's money and property. And Chapter 10 shows in detail the definite risks and potential benefits of private long-term care insurance—and explains the most important policy terms to consider.

■ *If your spouse or partner has personal assistance or medical needs the two of you are no longer able to handle without outside help, whether or not your spouse or partner has recognized the need:*

In Chapter 2, you will learn about how home care may permit you both to remain at home and get the care you need. Chapter 3 discusses the kinds of residential alternatives in which you might both live and receive the care you need with more comfort, but at much less cost than a nursing facility. Chapters 6 and 7 describe how the Medicaid government assistance program might help pay for one spouse's care while leaving the other spouse with some income and assets.

- *If you increasingly find that you cannot manage all your own personal or medical needs without outside assistance and you face an immediate need to organize long-term personal assistance or medical care:*

Extremely helpful and encouraging are Chapter 2 which introduces the many kinds of care available to you at home as alternatives to entering a nursing facility, and Chapter 3 which discusses the kinds of housing available for seniors that might provide the right level of assistance for you without the tremendous expense and unnecessary restrictions of a nursing facility.

C. Exploring Long-Term Care Options

Although the sudden onset of an illness or disability does not always permit much advanced planning for long-term care, this book encourages you to be the best comparison shopper possible. If you are able to explore alternatives before rushing into residence in a nursing facility, you improve your chances of obtaining the level of care you need, and perhaps saving a great deal of money.

Being prepared and researching alternatives when choosing long-term care allows you to realistically assess what is needed, and to choose only the kind of care that is actually required. In this way, you can avoid the loss of independence and great cost that come with taking on more care than is needed. This is particularly true when some combination of home health care and personal assistance is sufficient to permit a person to remain at home instead of entering a residential nursing facility. Or when an assisted living or residential care facility can provide sufficient care to allow a person to avoid entering a nursing facility. When time permits, certain financial planning you can do *before* residence in a nursing facility becomes necessary may permit you to protect some of the value of your home or life's savings.

Finally, but not least important, the more thorough you are, the greater the opportunity for everyone concerned to participate— particularly if the person who needs care is not easily able to investigate and make decisions on his or her own. With more alternatives, everyone involved will have greater emotional room to come to terms with the decisions to be made.

D. Recognizing and Discussing the Situation

If you are the one who needs care, you may find it hard to discuss it with others because it seems a blow to your self-esteem, a subject that means you are really "old." You may also be reluctant to begin a process of giving up some of your independence, and fearful of what it may mean to give up full control over your life. And when you know you need the help of your family, you may be reluctant to bring up the subject because you know it will mean adding burdens to their lives.

If you believe that someone else—a family member or other loved one—is in need of care, you may be reluctant to bring up the subject because it may seem like a challenge or an insult. And within the family there may be anxiety, guilt and wide differences of opinion about what care is needed and from where and from whom it should come. The first step in providing needed care is to overcome the reluctance to talk about it. Once the discussion has begun, the information in this book can be of great help in organizing and choosing the right kinds of care.

1. Getting Help From Others

To get discussion underway and onto the right track, it is often best to look outside the family. An unrelated person can sometimes soothe ruffled family feathers, present a neutral opinion and offer solutions not considered by the family. Also, it's sometimes easier to reveal fears and other feelings to an outsider than to an involved family member.

The following are some of the people you can turn to for help in beginning to evaluate long-term care needs:

- Your personal physician is often a good person to start with, not necessarily to moderate discussions but to give a prognosis of medical needs and to refer you to others who may be helpful in making plans.
- Traditional word-of-mouth is still one of the best ways to begin tackling any new problem. Friends and neighbors whose opinions you trust, and who may have already faced similar situations, are often a good source of information. So, too, the people at your local senior center may know of sources for long-term care assistance. These word-of-mouth sources often let you know of "unofficial" personal care aides who would not be available through more formal channels.
- A clergy member may be able both to help directly and to refer you and your family to professionals who can introduce alternatives and coordinate planning.
- County family service agencies, Area Agencies on Aging or other senior information and referral services are experienced sources that can provide direct access to specific care providers as well as

help you develop an overall care plan. These agencies can direct you to a counselor or social worker who specializes in long-term care for elders and who can help you begin your discussions and planning. (See the Resource Directory in the Appendix of this book.)

■ Once discussions are underway and residence in a nursing facility is not absolutely necessary, many people make use of the services of a professional geriatric care manager to see what at-home and other supportive services are available and to organize care from different providers. (Geriatric care managers are discussed in detail in Chapter 2.)

INVOLVE THE CARE RECEIVER

If you are a family member helping to plan for someone else's care, bear in mind that the most essential participant in planning long-term care is the person whose care is being considered.

---

2. Assessing Medical Needs

Because a specific physical or mental condition is often what leads to the need for long-term care, one of the first things to do is to get professional advice both about the need for immediate care and about likely changes over time. Your primary care physician is often the first person to talk with, although he or she may refer you to a geriatric specialist for further consultation.

An additional resource to help assess medical and personal care needs is a geriatric screening program. Local hospitals have them, as do community and county health centers. As with most initial referral questions, if you have trouble finding a geriatric screening program, check with the county social service agency, local or Area Agency on Aging, or call the senior referral number in the white pages of the phone book.

Some of the things that must be addressed when assessing an older person's need for medical care are:

Specific Medical Requirements

The doctor or other health screening personnel can discuss the elder's specific medical needs, such as monitoring and administering drugs, or providing physical therapy, explain what is involved in providing them and let you know who can do it. The doctor or health care worker can also discuss the level of ongoing care that would be required to deliver those medical services: family members supplemented by occasional visits from home care aides, a more sophisticated home care program, or various levels of residential nursing facility care.

Changes in Care Over Time

The doctor or other health care worker can also discuss the medical prognosis—that is, what the future is likely to hold: whether to anticipate a short or long recovery period, whether a condition is likely to remain fundamentally the same over a long period, or whether it will become worse over a short or long period. Knowing the likely developments in the medical condition will allow you to plan the right level of care and to allow for changes.

Mental Disabilities

A thorough geriatric screening and evaluation are particularly important when the need for care arises from what seems to be a mental impairment. An older person's physical problems may become much more difficult to manage because of added symptoms of forgetfulness, disorientation, or general listlessness.

Such changes are usually assumed to be the beginnings of a permanent loss of mental faculties: the early stages of Alzheimer's disease or other forms of dementia require careful long-term care planning.

Sometimes, though, what is thought to be an irreversible loss of mental facilities is really the result of some specific and treatable problem such as improper or over-medication, poor nutrition, depression about the loss of a spouse or a friend or about a physical disability, or a subtle medical condition that has not been diagnosed and treated. It is very important that a temporary and treatable loss of mental capacities is not misunderstood and perpetuated as a permanent condition.

In determining the true nature and cause of any loss of mental faculties, family members and friends can be particularly helpful to physicians and other health workers. The people who see an older person frequently are in the best position to know what factors may be contributing to diminished mental capabilities.

3. Assessing Personal Needs and Capabilities

Equally as important but usually more difficult than assessing medical needs is determining what sort of personal, non-medical care is needed and what aspects of daily life a person can still manage without outside assistance. The question of the need and ability to care for oneself is not simply a matter of physical competence. Often, it is just as much about personality and emotional state. So, in addition to what kind of care is needed and the providers who are available and affordable, the ultimate decisions should depend a great deal on how important it is to the elder to remain in control of his or her own life.

Some people fiercely hold on to personal independence and privacy. For these people, who also have the ability to organize, manage and pay for individual programs to meet their specific needs, staying at home and receiving only minimal outside assistance may be both possible and extremely important.

Others may be willing to have an outside agency organize a more comprehensive care program, as long as they or their family members remain in primary control of daily life. For these people, an agency-directed program of home care in a family residence or in secured housing, perhaps combined with adult daycare, may be most appropriate if there are also family members willing to give additional assistance.

Still other people, however, prefer the security and ease of complete care organized and provided by others. For them, a residential care facility may be best, even though they may not physically require the high level of care offered there.

4. Laws Providing for Family Leave

The first days and weeks during which a family member's need for long-term care arises can be extremely difficult and stressful. Balancing a job with your attempts to understand, locate and arrange care can be overwhelming. Temporary unpaid leave from work can be an enormous help during this period, but businesses have done poor jobs of providing family leave on their own.

In recent years, however, many states and the federal government have stepped in to mandate that employers provide some unpaid leave when a family member needs attention because of a health crisis. In particular, the 1993 federal Family and Medical Leave Act provides some needed help. Under the Act:

- Companies with 50 or more employees must give workers up to 12 weeks per year of unpaid leave to care for a child, spouse or parent with a serious health condition.

- Companies must allow employees to return to their old jobs, or equivalent jobs at the same pay, when they return to work.
- Companies must continue providing the same health benefits as when the employees are being paid.

However, there are some limits written into the law as well. Companies can limit medical leave benefits to employees who have worked there for one year at an average of 25 hours per week. And if companies doubt the medical need for the leave, they can obtain as many as three medical opinions and certifications on the medical need for the leave.

In addition to this federal law, some state laws are even more protective of workers, applying to businesses with fewer than 50 employees, and some providing longer leave periods. Some large companies also have their own leave policies which are more generous than state or federal laws require.

So, if you find that some unpaid time off work would help you organize long-term care for a spouse or parent, check your employer's policy and make sure it complies with federal law and the law of your state. And if, when you return to work after unpaid leave, you find that your job has been changed for the worse, you may be able to find legal recourse in your state law or the federal family leave laws.

Finally, if the family member who needs care has long-term care insurance, check the policy to see if it provides for respite care. Respite care pays for home care aides who give short-term breaks to family members who care for an elder. (See Chapter 10 for a discussion of long-term care insurance.)

E. Making a Realistic Family Commitment

The options older people have to receive long-term care while maintaining their independence often depend on the extent to which family members are able and willing to help. But family situations vary widely in terms of relatives who can provide care, transportation, companionship or financial support to an elder. Before any long-term care program is organized—particularly when the elder is to remain at home without a spouse—family members must get together and discuss what commitment each is willing to make to meet needs that cannot be met by outside care or which would be prohibitively expensive if provided by paid caregivers.

Some of the possible arrangements requiring different levels of family involvement are:

1. Staying at Home

The degree to which older people who need long-term care can maintain themselves in their own homes or apartments may depend on several kinds of family help. There may be a need for daily or weekly assistance with personal or medical care that is not provided by a home care or other outside agency. Help with housekeeping, shopping and home maintenance may be needed. And there will certainly be a need for regular visits and other help such as transportation to allow the elder to maintain contact with the outside world. Help may also be needed in planning, coordinating and overseeing outside care programs, as well as in planning and administering financial matters, including direct financial assistance.

2. Moving in With Family

If older people needing long-term care are unable to maintain themselves in their own homes, they may still be able to avoid the cost and loss of independence of a residential care facility by moving in with willing family members and receiving long-term home care there. This kind of arrangement may permit family members to supplement home care provided by outside agencies with direct care of their own, keeping down costs and keeping up personal control.

But such an arrangement is obviously not for every family. It requires sufficient physical space and financial resources. And it takes the willingness of both the elder and the relatives with whom the elder lives. Everyone involved has to give up some room and some privacy and must make adjustments in daily habits and expectations. Relatives with whom the elder does not live must also be willing to share the responsibilities: visiting, outings, financial assistance. Obviously, all this takes a lot of talking, planning and ongoing cooperation among all family members.

3. Entering a Residential Facility

Recent surveys of nursing facility residents have shown that contact with the world outside—leaving the facility for visits and outings, receiving visits, phone calls and mail from family and friends—is their single greatest concern. So even when an elder moves into an organized residential setting which provides personal care and social activities, or into a nursing facility which is supposed to provide complete care, family participation remains of the utmost importance.

To prepare for any residential care setting, family members must be willing to discuss both individually and as a group how much each is *realistically* able and willing to help. But most important, family members individually and collectively must discuss the future directly with the loved one who needs care.

F. The Ability to Pay

Most communities have a wide variety of home care programs and residential facilities, but almost all of them are quite costly. Home care is often much less expensive than residential care; part-time home care may run between $3,000 and $10,000 per year. But as more frequent and extensive home care is needed, it also becomes very costly: 24-hour home care with nursing may cost $100,000 per year.

Residential facilities vary greatly in cost, with independent living facilities beginning at around $20,000 per year, and the least expensive assisted living and residential care facilities running about $30,000. The average cost of a nursing facility is about $50,000 per year. And in each of these categories, the prices may reach $100,000 per year for some facilities—particularly those in urban areas.

Unfortunately, government programs and private insurance pay a much smaller chunk of these costs than most people think. Medicare pays only about 2% of all nursing facility costs, a limited amount for short-term home care and nothing at all for residential care except for short-term stays in skilled nursing facilities. (See Chapter 5 for a discussion of Medicare, medi-gap insurance and veterans' benefits.) Medicaid—or Medi-Cal in California—the federal program for low-income people, does pay about half of all long-term nursing facility costs and a significant amount of home care charges. But Medicaid will pay for these only after you have used up almost all your savings paying for your own care. And Medicaid pays nothing at all for assisted living or residential care facilities. (See Chapters 6 and 7.) Private long-term care insurance may pay some of the cost of nursing facility and home care costs, but often pays only a portion of the cost, and pays nothing at all for many types of residential care facilities.

A BRIEF LOOK AT MEDICARE, MEDICAID AND INSURANCE

Medicare. Virtually everyone 65 and over is eligible. Coverage for:

Home Care. Short-term only; skilled nursing and therapy but not custodial care

Senior residences (independent living). None

Personal care facilities. None

Nursing facilities. Skilled nursing facility only, following a hospital stay; full payment for only 20 days, partial payment for up to 100 days; only in facilities certified by Medicare

Medi-gap Insurance. Private insurance policies that can be purchased by individuals 65 or over. Coverage for:

Home Care. Some policies provide limited coverage for short-term care if Medicare also covers; no coverage for long-term care

Senior residences (independent living). None

Personal care facilities. None

Nursing facilities. Many policies cover short-term stays in skilled nursing facilities if Medicare also covers them, paying the amount Medicare does not; no coverage for long-term custodial care

Managed Care (with Medicare). HMOs or other managed care plans specifically for people on Medicare. Coverage for:

Home Care. Limited coverage for short-term care under Medicare rules; for extra premium, some plans offer extra home care coverage under easier rules than Medicare's; no coverage for long-term care

Senior residences (independent living). None

Personal care facilities. None

Nursing facilities. Short-term stays in skilled nursing facilities under rules similar to Medicare; no coverage for long-term custodial care

Medicaid (called Medi-Cal in California). Varies in each state; to be eligible, you must have very low income and assets, not counting home, car and household goods. Coverage for:

Home care. Personal as well as medical care; usually limited duration

Senior residences (independent living). Not usually any coverage

Personal care facilities. Coverage in some states for Medicaid certified assisted living and shelter care facilities; if covered, unlimited duration

Nursing facilities. Extensive coverage in facilities certified by Medicaid; no time limit

Long-Term Care Insurance. Private insurance policies; they vary greatly in coverage and amount of benefits. Coverage for:

Home care. Some policies cover only home care; more expensive comprehensive policies cover both home care and residential care; amount of coverage depends on amount of premium paid

Senior residences (independent living). None

Personal care facilities. Some policies cover long-term care in residential care (shelter care) or assisted living facilities if policyholder is unable to perform certain amount of activities of daily living

Nursing facilities. Coverage in licensed nursing and board and care facilities for custodial care if proven medically necessary or unable to perform activities of daily living; benefits depend on cost of policy and rarely cover full cost of care

1. Help With Paying

In many places throughout this book, you will see references to coverage, and lack of coverage, of long-term care costs by Medicare, Medicaid and private insurance. Chapter 5 is devoted entirely to Medicare, Medicare managed care and private medi-gap insurance coverage of long-term care; Chapter 6 covers Medicaid eligibility and coverage; Chapter 7 discusses how to protect personal assets and still qualify for Medicaid coverage and Chapter 10 covers long-term care insurance.

The chart on the previous pages presents a brief introduction to each of these subjects so that you will be familiar with them as you read through the first few chapters on long-term care alternatives.

2. Determining Income and Assets

The first step in assessing what money is realistically available for long-term care is to determine all income and available assets. For guidance, use the list that follows. Consider the last category—Liabilities—as a set-off to be subtracted from available financial resources. Since this listing is informal, for your own reference, precise figures are not important.

When you have a complete picture of income and assets, you may be able to take certain steps to protect some of those assets from long-term care costs. (See Chapter 7.)

When regular outside care does become necessary, determine which services and facilities might be at least partially covered by government programs or private insurance, and which are available at low or no cost.

Finally, involved family members must begin to think about their own financial contributions. While there may be no immediate need for money from relatives, the decisions made about long-term care may determine when money from beyond the elder's own resources will be required. The earlier this possibility is discussed, the easier it will be to plan and provide for it.

Here are the most common items and some that you might overlook when attempting to get a complete picture of your income and assets—an essential first step in making long-term care decisions.

INCOME AND ASSETS

I. Estimated Income

Ongoing business income
Social Security retirement or disability benefits
Pension benefits
Income from rental property
Income from patents or royalties
Other income

II. Liquid Assets

Cash
Savings and money market accounts
Checking accounts
Certificates of deposit
U.S. savings and other bonds
Gold, silver, rare coins and other precious metals

III. Personal Property Assets

Interest in ongoing business (ownership, stock option, profit-sharing)
Value of any patents or copyrights
Brokerage accounts and other stocks

Money owed to you
Automobiles, boats, other vehicles
Antiques and works of art
Valuable jewelry
Face value of life insurance
Miscellaneous

IV. Real Estate (full or partial interest)

Property #1 (principal residence)
Property #2
Property #3

V. Liabilities (what you owe)

Mortgage debts (all money you owe on real property listed above)
Personal property debts (loans)
Miscellaneous debts

GETTING AND STAYING ORGANIZED

As you fill out this list, you may realize that your financial and ownership documents may be located in a number of different places. If so, this is a good time to gather them together and put them in one safe place, then give a list of the documents and their location to family members or others you trust. *Nolo's Personal Recordkeeper* (Nolo) is a computer program and manual that offers assistance in gathering and organizing this information.

G. Help Getting Started: Geriatric Care Managers

In the last several years, a new and potentially helpful field has developed, known as private care management for the aging, or geriatric care management. Care managers are professional counselors or guides who, either on a one-time or ongoing basis, help assess long-term care needs and organize services to meet those needs. They can be particularly useful when family members live in a different city from the person who needs the care.

Geriatric care managers can assist with placement in different types of assisted living, residential care and nursing facilities. And they can be invaluable in guiding you through the maze of home health care and supporting services needed for long-term care in the home. Care managers are generally familiar with residential facilities and can match care needs with levels of care and ability to pay. They can evaluate home care agencies, and they may know of difficult-to-find services that may supplement care provided by an agency. They may also know of individual caregivers who can fill gaps in home care. One of their greatest services is to help set up a coordinated program of care among several providers. They also follow up, monitoring ongoing care and helping make changes as necessary.

However, despite a care manager's expertise, decisions about long-term care are too important to leave solely in the hands of any one advisor. You and other family members should consider and evaluate what a care manager recommends, meeting with all caregivers and visiting any residence the care manager suggests. You know best the abilities, needs and personality of the elder who requires care: the more you learn about long-term care choices and the more you participate in the decision-making process, the better able you will be to choose among the alternatives a care manager may offer.

1. Where to Find Geriatric Care Managers

As with other long-term care resources, your personal physician, a local senior citizens center, or friends and neighbors might be able to refer you to geriatric care managers.

You can also find geriatric care managers in the white pages of the telephone directory under "Geriatric Care," "Geriatric Management," "Older Adults Care Managers," or something similar. Your local senior information or senior referral directory—usually listed separately in the white pages (sometimes under county or city offices or public health department) can also make referrals. Several national organizations, including Aging Network Services, can help locate care managers in your area. (Addresses and telephone numbers for these organizations can be found in the Resource Directory in the Appendix of this book.) A national directory is available from the National Association of Private Geriatric Care Managers, 655 North Alveron Way, Tucson, AZ 85711, 601-881-8008.

2. Evaluating a Geriatric Care Manager

There is no easy way to know in advance whether a particular geriatric care manager is reputable and effective. Some care managers are connected to organizations dedicated to elder care; other excellent care managers, though, work on their own. Unfortunately, there are no firm guidelines and no state certifications yet for this relatively new field. Here are some ideas, though, on what to ask before hiring a geriatric care manager:

- Where has the care manager worked before? Experience with a local public agency that deals with the elderly is a good sign, as is work at a local nursing facility or home health care agency. Whatever the form, some public health experience is essential. The care manager should provide you with references from previous employment if you ask for them.

- What is the care manager's professional training? Normally, a care manager should have a license or degree in public health nursing, public health management, social work or gerontology. If not, be very sure that the person has an extensive work history you can check personally.

- Does the care manager belong to any state or national professional organizations? Membership in a professional organization such as the National Association of Social Workers, Visiting Nurse Association or National Association of Private Geriatric Care Managers does not guarantee quality of work, but it may indicate a professional attitude and a willingness to have credentials verified.

- How does the care manager structure fees? Find out in advance exactly what you will be charged for and how much. Some organizations operating with public or philanthropic support offer free or low-cost services to low-income individuals and families. With many private care managers there is a flat fee ($100 to $250) for the initial family visit and evaluation, then an hourly charge ($15 to $100) for making arrangements and for follow-up visits. Whatever the terms, make sure to get them in writing.

- How extensive is the follow-up? After initial arrangements have been made, to what extent is the care manager available for personal or telephone consultations? For emergencies? What are the charges? Are there continuing services available, such as weekly or monthly reviews or visits, either by phone or in person? And what happens if a service or provider the care manager has arranged for does not work out? On what terms will the care manager arrange for replacement services?

- Does the care manager have a business contract of any kind with a particular home care agency or residential facility? If so, you must be somewhat cautious about accepting the care manager's recommendation of that agency or facility; it may be influenced by the motive of steering business there. At least make sure that the care manager presents you with some alternatives.

■ Does the care manager have any clients or former clients who can give a personal recommendation? Speaking with someone who has used the care manager's services before may give you both confidence in the care manager and a better idea of what to expect.

USE ALL RESOURCES

Relying on a care manager should not stop you from also checking with friends and relatives or otherwise looking for care on your own.

H. Additional Considerations

The time when long-term care needs to be arranged is also a time to review other legal and financial matters. A person who needs long-term care may have increasing difficulty taking care of personal matters, so it is also a good idea to review legal and financial documents and arrangements. (Some of the matters to be reviewed are mentioned below, and are discussed more fully in Chapters 7, 8 and 9.)

1. Health Care Directives

When long-term care becomes necessary, it is a signal to prepare to make decisions about future health care choices. In particular, consider what kind of medical treatments you would like to receive if you become terminally ill or are in a permanent coma and are no longer able to communicate your wishes about your medical care. The options, procedures and documents vary a bit from state to state, but in most states, you need only fill out, sign and get witnesses for one or more simple documents entitled a Living Will, Directive to Physicians, or Durable Power of Attorney for Health Care. (See Chapter 8, Section A.)

2. Durable Powers of Attorney for Finances

Another concern you may have as you grow older is being assured that there is someone to make financial decisions in accordance with your wishes if you are no longer able to handle your financial matters on your own. A Durable Power of Attorney for Finances, which takes effect only if you become legally incompetent to handle your own financial decisions, may be a document you want to consider. This document can help ensure that your finances are handled as you wish, by someone you trust, and without the expensive, cumbersome and time-consuming process of going to court. (See Chapter 8, Section B.)

3. Wills

Although the need for long-term care usually does not mean that death is imminent, it may signal a decreasing competence to make decisions about income, assets and estate. It is a good idea to review any existing will—which may be years old and out of date—and to make a new will that meets with the current wishes of the person in need of long-term care. (See Chapter 9, Section A.)

However, if there is any question about an older person's mental competence to make a new will, or about whether that person might be unduly influenced by another person to make out a will in a certain way, it is best to consult a lawyer who specializes in wills and probate matters.

4. Living Trusts

The basic reason for creating a living trust is to keep assets within your control but to avoid probate and some death taxes after you die.

Some people have the misconception that living trusts also permit you to qualify for Medicaid coverage of long-term care. In truth, living trusts do not shield the assets in the trust when the government determines whether you are eligible for Medicaid to pay long-term care costs.

There is a special kind of trust which, under some very limited circumstances, might permit the trustmaker to qualify for Medicaid. Unfortunately, these trusts are very complicated and must be established more than five years before applying for Medicaid. (See Chapter 7.) You will probably require the advice and assistance of an experienced estate planning lawyer. (See Chapter 9, Section B.) ■

2

At-Home Care

Until recently, older Americans and their families had few choices when faced with elders' inability to care for themselves. The options were either family care at home or residence in a nursing facility or "rest home." Relying entirely on the family often placed an overwhelming burden on adult children and grandchildren and seriously strained family relations. Opting for care in a nursing facility, on the other hand, often created guilty feelings, seriously strained family finances, and at the same time restricted the elder's comfort and independence.

Fortunately, in recent years, a great increase in the number and kinds of home care services has meant that more elders who need care can either remain at home or live with relatives without putting undue stress on the family. The change has resulted in part from new technologies that make many medical treatments—such as oxygen and intravenous therapy—mobile enough for home administration.

Another impetus toward the home care option is the rapidly rising cost of residential nursing facility care, making consumers of medical care more interested in finding cost-effective alternatives. And in response to the larger number of people receiving medical care at home, agencies and programs have increased the kinds of therapeutic, nutrition, homemaking and other personal care services provided there.

This trend toward home care is particularly welcome given the fact that public health surveys indicate up to half of all nursing facility residents could live independently if they had adequate and affordable home care services. And other studies have shown that the longer people remain independent from institutional care, the better it is for their overall physical and emotional health.

Unfortunately, though, long-term home care is not always a practical solution. Home care may be sufficient and affordable if one needs help with some physical movements around the home— bathing and getting meals, for example—or with exercise or physical therapy or monitoring a chronic health condition. But if one needs extensive medical treatment, or close monitoring for many hours each day, the difficulty of arranging different types of care may make home care impractical—and the cost may become prohibitive. In most cases, long-term home care also requires family members who can fill in gaps that the outside care services do not cover. For many people without such family assistance, long-term home care is simply not an option.

HOME CARE NOW MAY STILL MEAN RESIDENTIAL CARE LATER

Even if home care is a workable alternative, it may not remain so. Physical needs change over time; home care that now works well may later become impractical. For this reason, you may want to begin planning for the possibility of residential care at some later date.

That planning should take two forms. First, get to know the kinds of residential facilities in your area. (Elder residences are discussed in Chapter 3, nursing facilities in Chapter 4.)

Also, begin to consider how you might pay for residential care. And if it appears that Medicaid may be an option, explore the ways that you may protect a certain amount of assets while still qualifying for Medicaid coverage. (Medicaid is explained in Chapter 6, asset protection in Chapter 7.)

A. What Is Home Care?

Home care encompasses a multitude of medical and personal services provided at home to a partially or fully dependent elder. Although home care is available for people of any age who require long-term care, this book focuses on the needs of older people. These services often make it possible for an older person to remain at home, or with a relative, rather than enter a residential facility for extended recovery or long-term care. In this book, the terms "home" and "home care" refer to the private house or apartment where the elder lives alone, with spouse or other family or friend.

Depending on what is available in your community, home care and related supplemental services can include:

- Health care—nursing, physical and other rehabilitative therapy, medicating, monitoring and medical equipment;
- Personal care—assistance with personal hygiene, dressing, getting in and out of a bed or chair, bathing and exercise;
- Nutrition—meal planning, cooking, meal delivery or meals at outside meal sites;
- Homemaking—housekeeping, shopping, home repair service, household paperwork;
- Social and safety needs—escort and transportation services, companions, telephone check, overall planning and program coordination service.

(See Sections C and D, below, for a complete discussion of the many available home care and related services.)

Not everyone using home care will need all of the services available, not every community will have every possible service and no single program or agency can provide everything that might be required. Additional needs may have to be filled by community agencies or organizations, adult daycare or senior centers, individuals hired through informal networks, family and friends. Complications caused by the special mix that each person needs—different services from different providers—is one of the reasons many people use a geriatric care manager to help establish a home care program. (See Chapter 1, Section G.)

1. Independence

One of the great advantages of home care is that it permits an older person to maintain a feeling of independence and comfort in a familiar home. Also, you and your family may be better able to control the care received and to avoid care that isn't needed or wanted.

On the other hand, for home care to work well, you and your family must take the initiative to find services, coordinate different programs and personnel, monitor home care needs and performance, figure costs and budgets and make changes when required. And the family will be making all these decisions without a professional institution to help. This decision-making responsibility can be a significant burden on top of helping to meet daily needs for physical care.

It is also true that for some people, remaining at home isolates them from social activity and limits mental stimulation. Although friends and family often intend to provide lots of companionship, too many elders wind up spending their days in bed asleep or watching television. An organized elder residence, on the other hand, offers both a community of people and a constant stream of activities.

2. Financial Savings

In addition to the physical and emotional advantages of remaining at home, there can also be significant financial savings if the care required is not too complicated or frequent and family and friends supplement paid care. While residential care facilities average $30,000 to $100,000 a year, home care can average from 25% to 75% less, depending on what care is required. You save by not paying for unnecessary services or institutional overhead. The things you provide yourself at home—food, drugs, supplies—come without any nursing facility mark-up.

However, home care that begins as cheaper than residential care often creeps up to become more expensive over time. Home care needs may become more extensive or complicated, and families may participate less, requiring paid help to fill in the gaps.

Or, it may simply be that hidden expenses wind up making the true cost of home care too high. Families often fail to calculate peripheral expenses: the continued or expanded cost of running a home such as taxes, utilities, insurance, maintenance; the cost to family members of transport to help care for the elder and the cost of missing work; the repeated costs of workers to supplement family and regular care.

3. Quality of Care

While the comfort and financial advantages of home care sound attractive, you may have some doubts about whether the quality of care at home is as high as in a nursing facility or other elder residence.

Medical and nursing care. The American Medical Association, the American Hospital Association, the American Nurses' Association and the U.S. Department of Health and Human Services all stand behind the quality of medical and nursing care delivered by home care agencies that are certified by both Medicare and your state's home care licensing agency. So, when medical or nursing care—as compared with assistance with non-medical activities of daily living—is a significant part of the home care you need, you may do well to concentrate on certified agencies rather than on independent caregivers. (See Section D.) It is also crucial to have your doctor participate in the decision about whether the medical or nursing care you require can be safely and adequately delivered at home.

Non-medical care. Most of the care people need at home is not medical or nursing care, but help with what are called the activities of daily living (ADLs). These include bathing, using the toilet, dressing, eating, getting in and out of bed or chair and walking around. For people with Alzheimer's or other cognitive impairment, home care may consist primarily of making sure that the person does not become lost, disoriented or injured. For these kinds of non-medical assistance, home care is often better than residential care. That is because home care is provided one-on-one, whereas residential facilities have staff-to-resident ratios of one-to-ten or more. And by choosing and monitoring a home care agency or individual home care providers, you may be better able to control the quality of care you receive. On the other hand, tracking the effectiveness of home care is primarily up to the family, whereas residential facilities have professional staff members who are supposed to check regularly on the quality of non-medical care provided.

B. How to Find Home Care Services

As you've probably gathered by now, arranging a program of home care involves some searching and organizing, and often means using services from more than one source. To do this, you need to learn where to find these services and how to locate recommended agencies and individuals.

Much of home care—particularly nursing and other medical services—can be provided by a home care or home health care agency. (The services such agencies provide are discussed below in Section C.)

There are a number of ways to find one:

1. Friends and Relatives

While the opinions of professionals are often helpful, friends and relatives who have had home care experiences can be an excellent place to start. Informal information-sharing can reveal a program or person unknown to an agency or professional, and can warn you about providers to avoid despite their apparently sound credentials. Call a few friends or relatives and tell them the kind of help you think you need. They may be able to tell you of other people they know who have arranged for similar help. This kind of networking can snowball, with each phone call leading you to others to contact for information or services. Don't be shy. Call around and start the snowball rolling.

2. Hospital Personnel

If you are looking for home care following a stay in a medical facility, most have a "discharge planner" or "social services" administrator who can refer you to a home care agency capable of meeting your needs. Many hospitals and skilled nursing facilities operate their own home health care units. Although you should not automatically sign up with the hospital or nursing facility's home care unit, it is a good place to start comparison shopping.

3. Physicians

Your own physician may know of a good home care agency with which he or she has worked. That would offer the assurance that your doctor is willing to work with the particular agency. Your doctor may also be willing to put you in contact with other patients who use the agency.

4. Nursing Registries

If your need is primarily for at-home nursing, contact your local hospital, which probably has a registry of visiting nurses. The local chapter of the Visiting Nurses' Association provides visiting nurses and may also be a good source of referrals for other care.

5. National, State and Local Agencies and Organizations

If your need for home care is the result of a particular illness or disability, ask for referrals from the local chapter of a volunteer organization that focuses on that illness or disability, such as the American Heart Association, American Cancer Society, American Diabetes Association, the Alzheimer's Foundation, among others.

Many public agencies that specialize in the needs of older people can also refer you to home care agencies in your area. The federal government has set up Area Agencies on Aging which operate some federally funded programs which can be of direct help; the area agencies can also refer you to Medicare-approved home care agencies.

Most states, too, have their own Agencies on Aging—and there may be local offices of the state agency in your own community. Check the state government listings in the white pages of the telephone book.

City and county Agencies on Aging may have low-cost programs of their own and can also refer you to reputable home care agencies. Referral services can be found in your phone book under listings for Senior Referral, Department of Social Services, Family Service Agency, or Information and Referral. Often these services have a social worker or public health worker who specializes in referrals for older people.

```
┌─────────────────────────────────────────────────┐
│              FOR MORE INFORMATION                │
│                                                  │
│  For addresses and telephone numbers of many of  │
│  these organizations and agencies, see the       │
│  Resource Directory in the Appendix of this book.│
│                                                  │
└─────────────────────────────────────────────────┘
```

FOR MORE INFORMATION

For addresses and telephone numbers of many of these organizations and agencies, see the Resource Directory in the Appendix of this book.

6. Senior Centers

Because it is part of the job of local senior centers to provide information for seniors, they are usually happy to help with referrals to agencies and individual services. Home care providers know that senior centers supply this information, so they often make their services known at the centers. You can also get personal recommendations and opinions from other older people at the centers.

7. Volunteer Organizations

A number of community volunteer organizations not only provide referrals, but also administer their own home care programs. Your local United Way, for example, is a good clearing house for different services. Churches or synagogues, and local religious, ethnic or fraternal agencies and organizations are often very helpful in coordinating home care services, usually free of charge, and in helping you make informal care arrangements.

OLDER PEOPLE HELPING OLDER PEOPLE

The Retired Senior Volunteer Program (RSVP) is a federally funded program through which retired older people volunteer to help other less mobile elders. RSVP, together with the Senior Companion Program, provides all sorts of general assistance with non-medical daily needs, free of charge. And if RSVP is not equipped to help you directly, it may well be able to refer you to a program or agency that can. To find your local RSVP, look in the white pages of the phone book under Retired Senior Volunteer Program or contact the national office of ACTION, 1100 Vermont Avenue, NW, Washington, DC 20525, 800-424-8867. The national office will help connect you with the branch nearest you.

C. Services Provided Through Home Care

Home care services range from highly skilled medical care, nursing and therapy to simple household tasks such as cleaning and cooking. And home care agencies can also provide what is called respite care, which is simply a stand-in home care provider who visits with an elder while a regular caregiver—usually a family member—takes a break or a respite.

1. Medical Services

Most home care agencies as well as Visiting Nurses' Associations can provide or arrange for a number of medical services, including skilled and basic nursing, rehabilitation therapies and dietary services.

Nursing

With a physician overseeing the course of treatment, a home care agency or nursing registry can provide geriatric nurse practitioners, registered nurses and licensed vocational or practical nurses. These highly skilled nurses plan and monitor health care, give injections and intravenous medication and instruct you on self-administered medications, injections and treatments.

More routine nursing care is provided by vocational and practical nurses and by aides who work under the nurses' supervision. They monitor pulse, blood pressure and temperature and administer simple diagnostic procedures, such as drawing blood and other samples for the laboratory and instruct home patients on how to use portable testing equipment.

Therapies

Most home care agencies provide a physical therapist, respiratory therapist, speech therapist or occupational therapist. These specialists give short-term assistance to people recovering from an illness or injury and ongoing therapy to those with permanent disabilities.

Nutrition

Most agencies also either have someone on staff or can arrange for someone to help plan a diet and show how to prepare foods that provide proper nutrition and meet special dietary needs. Help in shopping for and preparing meals may also be available, as are meals brought in fully prepared.

2. Medical and Safety Equipment and Supplies

Home care agencies can provide medical equipment and supplies such as a hospital bed, wheelchair, walker, oxygen equipment and various home testing and monitoring equipment, as well as supplies for incontinence and other conditions. The equipment can be either bought or rented from the agency or from a medical equipment company with which the agency does business.

Some home care agencies can also inspect your home for safety needs and arrange to install any necessary equipment, such as support railings, access ramps or an emergency response system.

ON SAVING MONEY

Find out whether you are required to buy or rent all medical equipment and supplies from any home care agency you are considering. If so, and you need substantial medical equipment or supplies, make sure their prices are competitive with what you would pay if you purchased the equipment or supplies on your own. Always comparison shop before buying equipment or having any work done through an agency.

---

3. Non-Medical Personal Care

Most people who consider home care do not need skilled medical care as much as assistance with personal tasks that have become difficult because of frailty or other physical debility. This is provided not by skilled medical personnel, but by "home health aides" or "home care aides."

Aides are the people who spend the most time with you. Their tasks vary, depending on your needs and on the rules of the agency or willingness of the individual aide, but in general they include:

- assistance with personal care such as bathing, grooming, toilet needs, eating;
- help with movement or exercise, such as getting in and out of a bed or chair, getting around the house, stretching, taking a walk;
- simple health tasks, such as taking blood pressure and temperature and helping with self-administered medications, salves and breathing equipment; and
- minimal homemaking, such as helping to plan and cook simple meals.

More general homemaking services (grocery shopping, meal preparation and clean-up, light housecleaning and laundry) are often available through home care agencies. Not every home care agency provides homemaking services, however, and you may need to make separate arrangements through informal networks of friends, relatives and neighbors or with an independent home care provider.

REMEMBER TO ASK

Just because something is not on a home care agency's or individual aide's list of offered services does not mean it is not available. Depending on how flexible your home care aide is, any light task around the house might be included. If the aide will not help, or is not allowed by an agency to assist with certain needed tasks, the agency may be able to provide someone who can.

Respite Care

With home care, the primary responsibility for care and companionship often still rests with family members. Particularly when an elder requires extensive monitoring, that can become a substantial burden on family members who must stay around the house. Some agencies provide temporary respite care—a companion for the elder, whose presence allows a family member to leave the house and go to work, attend to other business, or simply have a break. Obviously, you can also make private arrangements for someone to fill this need.

Respite companions are often volunteers, organized through a community group. If your agency does not have respite care, it should be able to refer you to a community group or organization that does provide it. (See Section J, Supplements to Home Care, below.)

D. Kinds of Home Care Providers

Home care providers range from hospitals or other high-tech organizations with highly trained medical staffs, to full-service home care agencies, to the ten-year-old kid down the block who takes out your trash. Getting the most sophisticated and well-equipped home care provider is not the point. The goal is to find providers who can bring you the specific care you need, and no more, for the best price.

1. Full-Service Home Care Agencies

Most home care agencies, whether their name refers to general home care or specifically to home *health* care, provide a great variety of services. Some agencies offer more services than others, although a few will supply all the services mentioned below. Some will help you find outside services they don't provide; others will leave it to you to fill in gaps. In any case, if there is a service you may need that the agency does not mention, be sure to ask about it. If an agency cannot provide the service, it may know someone who can. Many home care agencies will create a written care plan and provide a written estimate of costs as part of any contract you sign for their services. Review the care plan and contract carefully to make sure you are not obligated to buy, rent or pay for any services or equipment in the future.

Home care agencies are often affiliated with hospitals, nursing facilities and nursing organizations. But since most home care is *not* direct medical care, the fact that an agency is connected with a medical institution does not necessarily mean it will provide better overall personal care.

On the whole, full-service agencies tend to be more expensive than independent providers or support-care agencies that do not provide nursing or medical therapies. Despite their higher cost, though, they can be extremely useful when it is necessary to coordinate different levels of care and there are no family members available to organize and oversee separate independent providers.

2. Support-Care Agencies

Support-care agencies provide personal, household and respite care, but not skilled nursing or medical therapies. They are often sponsored by community or charitable organizations and because they do not maintain highly skilled medical staffs, some can provide home aides at lower rates than full-service agencies. (In choosing a support care agency, refer to the criteria discussed in Section E, What to Look for in a Home Care Agency.)

3. Independent and Informal Arrangements

As emphasized throughout this chapter, not all care must come through a formal agency. More important, not all *good* care comes from an agency. Independent home care workers are often more flexible in the tasks they will perform, and are also less expensive, than agency personnel.

Finding Independent Aides

Some communities have what are called In-Home Support Services that refer home attendants and aides for non-medical home care. And many public agencies, community or charitable organizations and churches, while not sponsoring a home care agency, offer a referral list of independent home care aides the organization or agency vouches for and has referred successfully in the past.

Professional nurses and nonprofessional aides can also be found through informal networks. Friends and relatives may know of an individual who suits your needs but who does not work through an agency and may not have any formal certification or training. Many people have found that "unofficial" aides provide very personal, flexible and competent assistance and charge considerably less than certified nurses or aides.

Keep in mind, though, that the range and quality of care you get depends entirely on the knowledge, skill and attitude of the one care-giver. There is no outside supervision, no one to compare the quality of care you are getting with the quality you should be getting. Also, with an independent aide, no agency has checked into the back-ground of the person who will be spending a considerable amount of time in your home. And while agencies routinely post a "bond" for their aides to protect the consumer from theft or damage by the home care aide, most independent aides are not bonded.

Finally, a common and significant problem with independent aides arises when they are sick or otherwise unavailable. If you will need an independent aide regularly, it is a good idea to have a back-up to call on short notice.

Home Care Personnel

Different types of care are provided by home care agency workers with different titles and skills. Knowing the types of personnel can help you make use of the services an agency has to offer. Also, because fees are higher for more skilled workers, understanding the different categories can help you avoid having an *overqualified*, and therefore overly expensive, home care provider when a less skilled but equally effective provider is also available.

Supervisors and Planning Coordinators. Probably the first person you will have contact with, the planner assesses your needs and capabilities and develops an overall plan for care. The planner may also oversee personnel assignments, and if so, may be the one to consult about changes in services or personnel after your care has begun.

Clinical or Nursing Supervisors. A clinical supervisor, usually a public health or geriatric nurse, monitors your direct home medical care, including diet and nutrition. This is the person for you, your family or your doctor to speak with if you have a question or problem with the skilled medical care you receive.

Social Workers. The agency's social worker, resource manager or caseworker can help coordinate your care with other programs and services not provided by the agency and can help with financial and insurance planning and paperwork.

Nurses. Every home health care agency should have at least one nurse practitioner or registered nurse (RN) on call at all times to monitor patient nursing needs. Nurse practitioners generally supervise other nurses, and can prescribe some medicines, give injections and diagnose routine medical problems. Registered nurses handle complex nursing functions, including administering intravenous medication, drawing blood and making an overall assessment of patient needs and a nursing care plan to meet those needs.

A Licensed Vocational Nurse (LVN) or Licensed Practical Nurse (LPN) handles the more routine nursing tasks, such as monitoring blood pressure and pulse, checking fluids, administering oxygen and some medications and doing some basic physical rehabilitation.

If you require a special physical rehabilitation program—after a hip injury or a stroke, for example—a Certified Rehabilitative Nurse (CRN) may plan the program, begin you on it and monitor your progress, sometimes in conjunction with a rehabilitation therapist.

Rehabilitation Therapists. Physical, occupational, speech and respiratory therapists plan and carry out a program of rehabilitative therapy. Once you are on a regular program, routine therapy assistance is often handled by trained assistants or technicians.

Home Care Aides. The home care aide is the foot soldier of home care. The aide handles simple, everyday health and personal care tasks: bathing, grooming, moving around, exercising, helping with self-administered medications, creams and therapies, monitoring blood pressure and temperature. The aide may also help you with minimal homemaking—planning and preparing simple meals, some amount of home organizing. But the home care aide is not a housekeeper or house cleaner; these services may or may not be available through your home care agency. An independent home care aide, on the other hand, may be more flexible about a certain amount of household work.

Companions. Sometimes the greatest need one has, particularly if house-bound, is simply for company. Some home care agencies provide, often through a community group, people known as "companions," who will spend time in the home or go for a small outing— shopping, to the library, to the park or just for a walk—to give an elder some company and conversation. Companions may also help with personal paperwork, make phone calls and organize slightly more complicated outings.

E. What to Look for in a Home Care Agency

Although you may find good quality and less expensive care without using a home care agency, if you do choose to use one, here are some of the things to look for:

1. Certification

This is not a guarantee of quality care, but a full-service agency should be approved by both Medicare and your state's Medicaid program. The government checks to make sure certain staff, supervision and basic training requirements are met. Likewise, if your state licenses home care agencies, make sure your agency has such a license. To find out, call your area or local Agency on Aging. (See the Resource Directory in the Appendix.)

Also, some agencies are accredited by national health care organizations. For example, the Joint Commission for Accreditation of Health Care Organizations is the umbrella organization that accredits home health care agencies.

2. Reputation

Here are some questions to ask:

- How long has the agency been in business? Look for an agency that has stood the test of time.
- Does the agency belong to the National Association for Home Care or to a state home care association? Membership may indicate adherence to certain standards of care.
- Can the agency give references to doctors and public health workers who have worked with the agency and to clients? Talk

directly with the references, and if medical care is involved, try to have your doctor do so, too.

3. Services and Flexibility

No matter how many services an agency claims to offer in its brochure, the important thing is to match its services with your needs. And if you have any special scheduling needs, make sure the agency will accommodate you. Also, find out if there is any extra cost for night or weekend services.

Flexibility in care is also very important. An agency may be able to meet your needs at first, but what if your needs change? Can the agency also provide different, more specialized medical services, a more unusual schedule, household work? It is not necessary that the agency *directly* provide every service you might need in the future, as long as it has the capacity to arrange the service through coordination with other providers.

Before choosing an agency, ask the planning coordinator about the availability of other services. What are their regular arrangements with other programs or agencies? What is the extra charge for such services? Can they arrange for services which they do not already have on call?

4. Personnel Standards

Find out about an agency's personnel before you begin to receive care. What are the skill levels of both in-home and planning personnel on staff? What training and experience are required for different positions? Even non-medical home care aides should have completed some formal training.

Since home care workers will be spending a significant amount of time in your home, often with no one else present, find out what process the agency uses to screen an employee's background.

5. What Does Not Matter in Choosing an Agency

Some things about home care agencies may seem to be important considerations in choosing a home care agency, but in fact are not important.

Nonprofit, Church-Related or Charitable Organization

Because an agency is "nonprofit," will it be less expensive? Or if the agency is sponsored or owned by a church or a charitable organization, will it have the client, rather than money or the appearance of doing good works, foremost in mind?

The answer to both questions is: not necessarily. Some organizations that operate home care agencies acquire nonprofit tax status by associating with a larger nonprofit group. This means they pay less in taxes, but it does not mean that the rates they charge will be cheaper; only a comparison of rates with other agencies can tell you that.

Nor does a nonprofit status mean the quality of care is any better. Just because a church or charitable organization sponsors an agency does not mean it has anything to do with the agency's daily operations. These are usually handled by an independent administration, and it is their work that determines the quality of care.

National Chain

An agency that is part of a large nationwide organization may appear to have a better administration than a small, independent agency. In

certain respects that may be true—for example, standardized personnel duties, or computerized billing may make some aspects of home
care easier to manage. But gains in paper efficiency may be lost in
personalized care. The quality of care you receive from any agency,
national chain or small independent, depends on the skill and attention of the people who will be in your home giving you hands-on
care.

Hospital-Connected

An agency affiliated with a hospital may appear better able to provide
medical care than other agencies. But keep in mind that most home
care does not involve complicated medical treatment. An agency that
focuses on high technology health care may be giving too little
attention to what most home care recipients need most—thoughtful
human attention.

F. Getting Started With Home Care

Whether or not you use the services of an agency, settling on a home
care plan is an important first step. Your diligence may also be required in supervising the care and updating the care plan as needed.

1. Developing a Care Plan

If you are using an agency, personnel there should consult with you
and your family in developing a plan, rather than imposing a pre-
arranged care package on you. Some agencies automatically deliver
more care than is needed, partly because the more services they

provide, the more money they make. Not only does this raise costs unnecessarily, but for many people, receiving too much care stops them from doing things for themselves, which can be an important part of continued psychological well-being. And agency or not, since your family will probably be providing additional care, family members should be directly involved in planning.

If you have special needs—rehabilitative therapy or restricted diet, for example—then specialists in those areas should also participate in planning. And consultations with your doctor should also be a part of the development of a care plan. It is important for a home care plan to take into account your overall comfort and need for human contact as well as specific medical care—for example, providing aides who can speak a language you are comfortable speaking, or aides who do not smoke, if that is your preference. In search of such a match, an agency planner should make at least one extensive visit to the home where you will be receiving care *before* finalizing a plan. And although you will certainly be keeping an eye on your own financial limits, an agency planner should also take into account your financial capabilities.

If you are making up your own care plan, it may help you keep track by using a checklist such as the one below. Be sure to include family members and friends who will help with care as well as paid or volunteer outside aides.

CHECKLIST FOR HOME CARE PLAN

1. Medical and Rehabilitation Care:
    Service:
    — Provider:
    — When provided:
    — Additional non-professional:
    — Follow-up care (who & when):
    Service:
    — Provider:
    — When provided:
    — Additional non-professional:
    — Follow-up care (who & when):
    Service:
    — Provider:
    — When provided:
    — Additional non-professional:
    — Follow-up care (who & when):
2. Non-medical Care (including personal assistance, meals, homemaking, escort, companion, transportation, phone check):
    Service:
    — Provider:
    — When provided:
    Service:
    — Provider:
    — When provided:

---

2. Getting Regular Providers

A home care plan is only as good as the people who carry it out. In addition to the training and experience of home care personnel, something harder to evaluate—how well you get along—is also important. It helps to meet and interview home care aides before they begin to provide care. Although it can save everyone trouble later on, some agencies discourage advance selection to prevent clients from overshopping for the "perfect" aide.

Continuity of care givers is also important. Once you have developed a relationship with care givers who understand your needs, you want to be able to count on them regularly. On occasion, there are legitimate reasons, such as illness or vacation, for a temporary substitute. But even in these instances, substitute care should be provided only by an aide regularly employed by the agency and not by an independent or "freelance" care giver unless that person's qualifications and background have been subjected to the same scrutiny as regular employees.

3. Supervising and Reviewing

If you use the services of a home care agency, that agency should regularly review the care plan. The original plan may not have addressed your needs adequately, your needs may have changed over time, or the people actually giving you care may not be doing their jobs properly.

A staff member skilled in the specific care involved should regularly supervise and review your care. A certified therapist should be checking on your therapy aide and a registered nurse should be checking on health care aides. The frequency of the reviews depends on the level of care. Medicare, for example, requires that a supervisor visit the home *at least every two weeks* if the care is for a chronic or acute illness. If there is no skilled medical care involved, home visits by supervisors can be less often—every four to eight weeks, perhaps—but a supervisor should be in at least weekly contact with the care giver.

There should be an easy way for you to register complaints with a supervisor about the care you are receiving. There should be frequent telephone contact between you and a supervisor, and there should also be regular in-person supervisor reviews of your care—with your family members present, if you wish.

G. Costs of Home Care

As discussed in Chapter 5, you cannot count on Medicare, medi-gap health insurance or managed care to pay for much of the costs of long-term home care. Medicaid (Medi-Cal in California) will pay for long-term home care, but only if you have little income and have used up most of your own assets. (See Chapter 6.) Even if you have long-term care insurance coverage for home care, it will probably pay only a portion of your total home care costs. (See Chapter 10).

Since you are likely to have to pay for most long-term home care costs out of your own pocket, pay close attention to the way a provider—particularly a home care agency—calculates its charges. Many agencies will give you a written estimate of charges based on the care plan they develop with you. Before signing up, read the estimate carefully, making sure it does not include charges for services you do not need or want. And after you have been receiving home care for a while, check the agency's bills against the estimate and compare the services for which you are billed with the services you are actually receiving.

GOVERNMENT-CERTIFIED PROVIDERS

Medicare and Medicaid approved. Even if the care you receive initially is not covered by Medicare or Medicaid, or you are not eligible for Medicaid, make sure an agency you use is certified for both. Your physical situation may change, making your care eligible for Medicare coverage. (See Chapter 5.) Or your financial situation may change, making you eligible for Medicaid. (See Chapter 6.) If the agency is certified, you would be sure of continuity in your home care.

State licensed. Some states have minimum quality standards and issue home care licenses or certificates to those agencies or individual providers that qualify. If you have private medigap insurance, Medicare managed care or long-term care insurance that covers home health care, it usually requires a state-licensed provider. (Medi-gap and managed care coverage of home care is discussed in Chapter 5, long-term care insurance in Chapter 10.)

---

1. Sliding Scale (Income-Based) Fee Policy

Many public agency, community, church and philanthropic organization home care providers base eligibility and fees on the care recipient's income. In other words, you only qualify if your income is below a certain level and the lower your income, the lower the charge. These are not always full-service home care agencies, but if they can meet your needs, they may offer significant savings for you.

2. Cost Varies With Service and Skill Level

Most agencies and individual providers charge by the hour or by the visit. Agencies sometimes also have a minimum daily or weekly charge. Generally, the amount charged reflects the skill level of the provider. It therefore makes sense not to receive simple care from a highly skilled provider when someone less skilled can provide it just as well. Roughly, rates are divided as follows:

- nurse practitioners and registered nurses, $50 to $100 per hour
- practical and vocational nurses, licensed rehabilitative therapists and geriatric social workers, $35 to $75 per hour
- home health aides, $10 to $20 per hour
- homemakers, home workers and companions, $7 to $15 per hour

Note. The rates charged by independent care givers are usually lower than those charged by agencies. The rates also vary in different parts of the country.

3. Beware the Hidden Charges

When you discuss rates with a prospective home care agency or other provider, make sure to find out about possible hidden charges. For example, there is sometimes a minimum charge per visit, per week, or per month. There may also be higher rates for night and weekend care, which could mean a significant cost increase if you require such care. So, too, some agencies charge extra for in-home assessments, evaluations and for visits by supervisors. These last are necessary elements of overall home care planning and service, however, and should *not* be charged as "extras."

HELP WITH HOME CARE COSTS

Medicare, Medicaid, medi-gap, managed care, long-term care insurance. All these programs and insurance coverage pay some of the cost of home care. Unfortunately, only Medicaid pays the full cost of long-term care.

Medicare. Pays for short-term home health care—a week up to a couple of months—but not for long-term care. Pays for home care only if you need skilled nursing or rehabilitation. (See Chapter 5.)

Medi-gap insurance & Medicare managed care plans. Medi-gap policies pay nothing for long-term home care. The same is generally true for Medicare managed care plans, although a few managed care plans offer some extra home care coverage for an extra premium. (See Chapter 5.)

Medicaid. Pays for long-term home care by certified providers. You may qualify only if you have very low income and assets. (See Chapter 6.)

Long-term care insurance. Some long-term care insurance policies cover home care. Payments begin only when you meet their benefit standards—meaning that, according to their rules, you need the care. (See Chapter 10.)

H. Financing Home Care Through Reverse Mortgages

An older person who has very low income and few assets may qualify for Medicaid, which can pay for the entire cost of home care. (See Chapter 6.) Or, an elder may have a long-term care insurance policy that will pay a portion of home care costs. (See Chapter 10.) However, many older people are caught in the middle. They have no long-term home care insurance coverage, they do not have enough income or liquid assets to pay for the long-term home care they need, but they do not qualify for Medicaid coverage.

Many of these same people, however, own their own homes or condominiums outright, or have considerable equity in them. And recently a mechanism has been developed that can convert home equity into cash for older homeowners while permitting them to continue living in the home as long as they are physically able to do so. This mechanism is called the "reverse mortgage"—basically, a loan against the value of a home which pays a lump sum, monthly amount or line of credit or some combination and does not require repayment until the borrower either sells or otherwise permanently leaves the home.

Reverse mortgages also have a side benefit. Because the money they provide is a loan, it is neither taxable income nor does it count as income against Social Security benefits if you are under age 70. The interest you accumulate on the loan, however, is not tax deductible until the loan is paid off.

When the borrower sells the home, he or she must pay back the loan out of the proceeds. If the borrower permanently leaves the home—moves in with relatives, to a nursing facility or other location—or dies, the lender must be repaid within a certain time, usually one year to eighteen months. This often means that once the borrower has left the house, it must be sold by the borrower or the estate to repay the reverse mortgage. The final amount of the repayment is determined by the size of the loan, the interest rate, the cost of insurance and the length of time the loan is outstanding.

If the amount paid on the reverse mortgage, including interest, is less than the amount for which the property is eventually sold, then the owner or owner's survivors keep the difference. If, on the other hand, the amount paid to the property owner under the reverse mortgage is more than the sales price, neither the owner nor the survivors owe the mortgage company anything more; the mortgage company has to take the loss.

There are several types of reverse loans and mortgages, each with somewhat different terms and purposes.

Property tax deferral programs. On a small scale, there are publicly funded and operated property tax deferral programs available in many states. These programs defer for low-income elders the value of their property tax and take a lien for the amount against the property, payable when the elder leaves the home and it is sold. Although these deferrals are for relatively small yearly amounts, they free up some cash for home care or other needs which would otherwise go to property taxes. For information about whether such a program is in place where you live, contact your county property tax collector or your Area Agency on Aging, or call your local Senior Information and Referral number in the white pages of the telephone directory.

Deferred home improvement loans. Some state and local government agencies also make loans to low-income elders to repair or improve their homes, with repayment deferred as long as the elder continues to live in the home. Although these loans are for limited amounts and specific purposes, they can help finance necessary improvements on a home, either to fit it specially for assisted living or merely to repair it so it remains livable. And this money an elder gets to make home improvements can free up other money for use on home care services.

HUD-insured reverse mortgages. The federal Department of Housing and Urban Development (HUD) insures some reverse mortgage loans through its Home Equity Conversion Mortgage (HECM) program; the loans are processed through private lenders and are available to any homeowner age 62 or older, regardless of his or her income. The loans are available to any owner or occupant of a single-family primary residence—including condominiums, but excluding co-ops and motor homes.

Privately insured reverse mortgages. In addition to HUD-insured loans, certain private mortgage holding companies also insure reverse mortgages administered by local lending institutions. These loans have less stringent qualifying standards and higher equity limits than HUD-insured loans, but they also charge higher fees and interest rates.

1. Drawbacks of Reverse Mortgages

Although reverse mortgages present some attractive features, they may also have some serious drawbacks. They often have high initial fees such as appraisal fees, credit checks, insurance, closing costs, origination costs and service charges. So, if you die or move out of the home without having drawn much on the mortgage, you wind up paying a very high cost for what will have turned out to be a short-term loan.

And there are continuing fees and interest payments each year, which may take a serious bite out of the money you actually receive. When considering any reverse mortgage, have the lender show you in writing exactly what these Total Annual Loan Costs (TALCs) will be, not just for the initial year, but for the entire life of the loan.

Even more significantly, interest under a reverse mortgage loan compounds; in other words, you wind up paying interest on interest as the loan period goes on. In addition, as more is borrowed monthly or under a line of credit, the principal also goes up. The combination of these two spiraling debt factors is that over a period of years, a modest initial reverse mortgage can cost considerably more than more conventional forms of borrowing and can eat up all the equity in the property. And an elder who wants to preserve some equity to pass on to heirs or to use in some other way after selling the house may very well wind up instead having a piece of property with no residual value.

Also, a reverse mortgage ties the borrower to the house. Most reverse mortgages require that the loan be repaid when the borrower no longer lives in the house. If the borrower decides to move in with relatives, or move to another area, or enters a nursing home to receive better care, monthly payments and any line of credit stop—and the borrower must repay the loan within a certain time. Elders who borrow under reverse mortgages may one day find themselves faced with the unhappy choice of moving to a more comfortable, healthy or secure setting, but ending loan benefits and having to pay off the loan, or continuing the mortgage benefits but staying put.

2. Protecting Your Interests

There are several things that people who shop for a reverse mortgage should insist upon to protect themselves and their home equity.

First, the mortgage must have a "nonrecourse" clause. This means that the lender has no recourse to any source of debt repayment other than the house. This limits the debt—no matter how long the borrower lives, how high the interest payments pile up or how many other assets the borrower has—to the value of the house.

Second, do not consider any reverse mortgage that requires you to transfer title to your property or to transfer title out of your name. A reputable reverse mortgage is a loan with an interest in your equity, not a transfer of title.

Third, never pay any application or processing fees until you have actually decided to apply for a specific loan. If a company tries to get you to pay before you even try to enter a contract with them, you can be sure it will try unfairly to squeeze money from you all the way down the line.

All HUD-insured loans require that a potential borrower receive counseling from a financial adviser unconnected to the lending institution. This adviser can explain all aspects of the loan and highlight its advantages and disadvantages. If you are considering a non-HUD loan, follow the same procedures. Consult with an independent financial adviser unconnected with the institution offering you the reverse mortgage, and discuss in detail all of the mortgage's benefits and risks.

For information on where to locate reverse mortgages and how to evaluate the ones being offered, see the Resource Directory in the Appendix at the end of the book.

I.   Cashing in a Life Insurance Policy

For many people who are nearing the end of life, being able to remain at home rather than entering a care facility may be very important. But the level and frequency of care required to keep a terminally ill older person comfortable at home may not be affordable. If a terminally ill person has a life insurance policy, however, it may be possible to use the policy to get a substantial amount of cash before death rather than waiting for it to pay after death.

However, there are potential consequences to cashing in a life insurance policy that may make the option somewhat less attractive than it first appears. First and most obviously, the policy benefits will no longer go to the original beneficiaries. And the benefit amount will be considerably lower than its face value, which is the amount that would be paid after death. Also, the payments may be subject to state capital gains tax; the federal government exempts these amounts from taxes, but some states consider them taxable income. This potential tax consequence, plus the complicated terms of the settlements themselves, make it important to consult with a financial advisor before entering an accelerated benefit or viatical settlement agreement. (See Section I2, below.)

Perhaps most significantly, the amount received may disqualify the elder from receiving Medicaid coverage for home or nursing facility care. (See Chapter 6.) Medicaid does not consider the face value of a life insurance policy as an asset, and does not require a Medicaid applicant to cash in a policy. But if a policy is cashed in, Medicaid will count the money received as an asset. And if the benefits push the elder over the Medicaid eligibility limits, cashing in the policy will have created a double loss: the elder won't qualify for Medicaid coverage and the policy will have paid much less than its face value.

For many terminally ill people, however, the benefits of getting the cash clearly outweigh these negatives. If getting the money before death seems worth it to you, there are two avenues for selling or exchanging a life insurance policy: through accelerated or living benefits and viatical settlements.

1. Accelerated or Living Benefits

Some life insurance policies may be cashed in directly with the insurance company itself—a procedure known as collecting accelerated or living benefits. The amount of these benefits runs between 60% and 80% of the face value of the policy, depending on the terms of the particular policy. If the policy provides for accelerated benefits, it usually requires that the treating physician must declare the policyholder terminally ill—meaning that he or she has less than two years to live.

The procedures by which to claim accelerated benefits are determined by the terms of the individual policy. To learn whether a policy may be cashed in for accelerated benefits, and how that process works, check the terms of the policy and speak with a representative of the insurance company that issued it. Do not rely on an insurance agent to explain the details; ask to be referred to staff that specializes in accelerated benefits.

2. Viatical Settlements

Even if a life insurance policy does not provide for accelerated benefits, a similar result may be achieved by selling the policy to a viatical settlement company. These companies take over as beneficiaries under the policy, meaning they get to collect the full face value when the policyholder dies. In exchange for that right to collect later, the settlement company provides cash at once: 60% to 80% of the policy's face value, depending on the length of the policyholder's life expectancy; the longer the life expectancy, the less they pay.

As with accelerated benefits, a policyholder must have been diagnosed to be terminally ill to qualify for a viatical settlement. But unlike accelerated benefits, the policyholder must also obtain written permission from the existing beneficiaries.

To shop for the best viatical settlement, compare at least two or three companies. Begin with your own insurance agent or one of the organizations that monitor viatical companies. (See the Appendix at the end of this book.) Regardless of how you find a viatical settlement company, check with your state's Department of Insurance to make sure the company is licensed to do business in your state; a state license at least means that the company's business practices are subject to some official oversight.

HURRY UP AND WAIT

If you cash in a life insurance policy, it usually means that you need the money immediately. But take the time to consider several companies, to compare all the options offered and to carefully review all the paperwork before deciding on a settlement. It might also be a good idea to consult with an accountant, lawyer or other financial advisor. And be aware that the insurance and viatical settlement companies also take their time considering your application and plowing through their bureaucratic steps before any money actually changes hands. Expect the entire process to take two to four months.

J. Supplements to Home Care

Along with the growth of home care, a number of free or low-cost programs now provide older people with certain services not offered by most agencies. These programs add to the home care services, keep costs down and often make the difference between being able to stay at home and having to enter a nursing facility. Most of all, many of these services give the person receiving care a break in the routine and give family members some relief from their responsibilities.

1. Meals-on-Wheels

Meals-on-Wheels is perhaps the best known supplement to home care. Although good nutrition is essential to health, many older people begin to neglect their diets when shopping, cooking and cleaning become difficult, or when dietary problems restrict food choices. Meals-on-Wheels brings easily affordable food that is hot, tasty, nutritious and ready-to-eat. It also provides daily, friendly human contact that is a welcome diversion in a long day at home.

Almost all communities now have some kind of low-cost meal delivery system for housebound elders, although in some areas there is a waiting list for this service. Funding for Meals-on-Wheels varies, and the service often depends heavily on volunteers, but all of the programs work essentially the same way. For a very small fee, Meals-on-Wheels delivers a hot, nutritional meal once a day, usually around lunchtime. Often, for a slight extra charge, you can also have a snack or another meal, either cold or easily heated, for later in the day.

2. Adult Daycare and Respite Care

Adult daycare can be either a supplement to home care or a virtual substitute for it. In general, adult daycare centers operate during daytime work hours and provide a meal, monitoring and companion-ship for people who need some care but are not seriously ill or disabled. Respite care provides a few hours a week of low-cost or free companionship without any active care services. Daycare centers and respite care are often funded by nonprofit organizations, and the programs that do not provide medical care tend to be less expensive than home care.

Adult Daycare Centers

Adult daycare centers provide different levels of medical care and therapy, along with meals, companionship, activities and social services. They offer family care givers who work an alternative to using full-time providers at home. For those receiving the care, they can often make the difference between living at home or entering a nursing facility.

Centers affiliated with a hospital or nursing facility may offer extensive medical care—including administering medications and treatments, monitoring specific conditions, health testing and preven-tive screening—all in keeping with a written, regularly revised health care plan. Rehabilitative therapies should also be available. A physi-cian should be on call and an RN or nurse practitioner available at all times. At centers run by community or public service organizations, less comprehensive medical care may be available.

Participants in adult daycare may stay for a half or full day, one to five days a week; regular, scheduled attendance may be required. Costs depend on the range of services offered and the nature of the sponsoring organization. Many charge according to the ability to pay. If transportation is not provided by the center, the center will often arrange for it.

In addition to medical services, adult daycare centers provide meals and snacks, personal care assistance, exercise, recreation and outings and social and educational programs. Also, social services, including referrals to other agencies and programs, are usually available. Above all, adult daycare centers offer companionship for elders who might otherwise be housebound.

FINDING ADULT DAYCARE

If you have difficulty finding an adequate adult daycare center, to get a referral and references for a center nearby contact:

National Adult Day Services Association
600 Maryland Avenue, SW, West Wing 100
Washington, DC 20024
202-479-6682

Respite Care

Like adult daycare, respite care serves as a break in routine for both those who give and those who receive care. Unlike adult daycare centers, however, respite care does not involve organized activities or services. It provides companionship and monitoring, often by volunteers, for short periods of time on a regular or occasional basis—a few times a week, one weekend a month, or for a full weekend or week when primary care givers are unavailable. Respite care can be provided at home (yours or the care giver's), at a church or community center, or in a nursing facility. It is often sponsored by a community organization and, unless it is at a medical facility, is usually low-cost or even free.

3. Senior Centers

Most senior centers provide free social and recreational activities, education, information and exercise programs and a hot meal on a drop-in basis to physically self-sufficient elders. Generally, there is no fixed schedule required for participation, although meals and some programs may have to be signed up for in advance.

While senior centers do not offer personal assistance care, they do provide some respite care, nutrition, organized activities and informal companionship for an elder who does not need monitoring. Senior centers often arrange for transportation to and from the center and sometimes organize outings to places of interest. They are excellent sources of information about services available to seniors, particularly about the individual, independent care givers who can be reliable and less expensive alternatives to agency care but who are sometimes difficult to find.

4. County Health Screening

One of the functions of skilled home health care is to monitor the health of the elder receiving care. If you require less attentive care, however, you may be missing regular health monitoring and screening. As a supplement to doctor visits, many city or county health clinics regularly offer free or low-cost health screening and testing. These clinics can provide adequate general health monitoring if used as part of an ongoing care plan. The public health nurses at these clinics can help schedule a regular program of screening and testing.

5. Family Education Programs

A number of public agencies and community organizations—United Way, Red Cross, Visiting Nurses' Association and many hospitals—offer instruction for elders and their families on various aspects of home health care: personal care assistance, such as bathing and movement techniques; exercise; nutrition for special dietary needs; monitoring health conditions and vital signs. Learning these techniques helps assure the safety and well-being of the elder and permits family members to assist with a wider range of home care—avoiding some of the dependence on professional providers. A family education program can also be a good source of information about other available programs, as well as a chance to share information and experiences with other elders and their families.

6. Additional Services

In addition to the programs discussed above, there are other specific services available free or at very low cost which can help lighten the burdens of home care.

You can find services to supplement home care much the same way you find home care itself. With supplemental care, however, the referrals are more likely to come from local rather than state or regional agencies, and from volunteer and community organizations rather than from institutions or medical sources. The local senior center is usually an excellent source of information, as is the Senior Referral telephone service listed in the white pages of your phone directory. Geriatric case managers can be particularly helpful in finding the small, independent or little-known extra services not provided by home care agencies.

Some of the supplemental services available in many communities are:

Senior Escort Service

Some people can get around on their own, or with minimum assistance, for short trips to the store or the bank or the park, for example, but are concerned about their safety on the streets. Escort services provide someone to accompany you on short trips; they're often available on fairly short notice.

Transportation Service

Many people would make trips to a senior center, the library, a park, or to organized activities if only they had the transportation. There are a number of public agencies and community groups that provide free transportation, often with wheelchair access.

Companion Service

Similar to respite care, a companion service can send someone for a few hours a week on a regular schedule, to provide company but not care. The occasional company and conversation of someone who brings good cheer can be a wonderful diversion. These services are mostly volunteer-staffed and community-funded, so there is usually no charge for using them.

Housekeeping and Grocery Services

Many state and local government Departments of Social Services or volunteer programs offer grocery shoppers and part-time housekeepers to do occasional work for low-income physically disabled or impaired elders. When available, these housekeeping and grocery services are offered free or at a very low cost.

Telephone Safety Service

Particularly valuable for people who live alone and who do not have family in the vicinity, telephone reassurance programs provide a daily call, at the same time each day, to make sure an elder at home is doing all right. And besides being a safety check, it is always nice to have a brief conversation with someone during the day.

A related service, called Lifeline, is available in many places and provides a telephone emergency response service usually connected directly to a hospital or other emergency health facility. The line can be connected to your phone and maintained for a nominal cost. ■

Organized
Senior Residences

Many seniors are no longer able, or no longer willing, to live completely independently at home. For some, home care may offer help, but it may not deliver the sense of security and companionship that is needed. For seniors at the other extreme, the amount of home care they need may make it too expensive, but they may neither want nor need the institutional care of a nursing facility.

Elder residences have evolved to fill this gap. They combine some of home's comforts and independence with some of the care and security of a nursing facility. The residences come in various shapes and sizes, provide different services and levels of care and carry different price tags. But they share at least one thing: they provide shelter and services for the elderly without the institutional feel and high cost of nursing facilities.

These organized residences range from seniors-only apartment complexes and retirement communities for relatively independent elders, to assisted living facilities for people who need help with activities of daily living. Some residential communities offer both independent living and assisted living in the same location. Still others provide continuing care, which includes a nursing facility and guarantees that a resident may move from one level of care to another as needed.

While organized senior residences may provide excellent living situations, they are not for everyone. Some facilities deny entry to seniors who are over a certain age, while others mandate a certain level of physical capability. And most are quite expensive. The exception is federally subsidized housing for low-income seniors, which may charge rent and provide some services on a sliding scale based on income.

And financial assistance is hard to come by. Medicare, Medicaid and private insurance do not cover any of the cost of independent living residences. Nor do they pay for most assisted living facilities, although this is slowly changing. (See Section B.) Nonetheless, most of the residential alternatives discussed in this chapter are less expensive than nursing facilities and are worth considering if some care, but not a nursing facility, is needed.

HELP IN FINDING RESIDENTIAL FACILITIES

A growing number of sources offer help in finding suitable residential facilities.

- American Association of Homes and Services for the Aging can provide you with information about its member residential facilities in your area. Phone: 800-675-9253; Internet: www.aahsa.org.
- Assisted Living Federation of America provides a list of assisted living facilities that belong to the federation. Phone: 703-691-8100; Internet: www.alfa.org.
- Your local Area Agency on Aging provides information about subsidized housing and residential facilities. (See the Appendix for contact information.)
- The Senior Referral and Information service listed in the white pages of the telephone directory can refer you to local facilities.
- A geriatric care manager may be able to direct you to residential facilities, might know the reputation of particular local residences and can help you evaluate whether a particular place is likely to meet your needs. (See Chapter 1, Section G.) A geriatric care manager may be especially useful regarding assisted living facilities.
- Religious, ethnic or fraternal organizations are often a good source for information about senior housing.

A. Independent Living

Independent living complexes are housing built or renovated for older people who are, for the most part, able to care for themselves. The main purpose of these residences is to provide senior-friendly housing and social services.

IF MORE CARE IS NEEDED

Independent living residences do not provide personal care or monitor a resident's physical condition. But some include separate floors or wings with assisted living units where such care is provided. (See Section B.) In these facilities, a resident may move to a higher level of care when needed, but only if such a housing unit is vacant. (See Section C1.)

Other independent living residences are combined with both assisted living and a nursing facility. In these continuing care communities, residents are guaranteed whatever level of care they need. (See Section C2.) If health or physical condition changes, a resident may move to a different level of care without having to wait for available space. This guarantee makes continuing care communities more expensive than multi-level facilities that permit a change only if there is a vacancy.

---

1. The Basics

Independent living residences come in many forms. For people with a good deal of money and independence, there are luxury, gated housing developments, often with a golf course or other extensive indoor and outdoor recreation amenities. In these developments, people purchase their own homes or townhouses.

There are also more moderately priced rental apartment or condominium complexes with a selection of differently sized units, common dining and socializing areas and services for residents, but without the extensive private grounds and recreation facilities of gated communities.

Independent living residences may also be simple urban apartment buildings with small rental units, limited common areas and few services. Some of these senior apartment buildings are subsidized by the federal government, meaning that rent is considerably cheaper than market rates for units of the same size.

Many independent living residences refer to themselves as communities. This may seem like a big claim for what may be no more than a small apartment building, but a sense of community is just what these residences seek to create. The amount and type of services offered by an independent living facility vary, depending in large part on cost. But all independent living residences provide a specially tailored and protected living space—a community—by:

- limiting residence to seniors, which means the people who live there tend to have similar experiences, physical capabilities and limitations
- designing and outfitting common areas and individual living units specially for elders, with elevators, ramps, wide hallways, good lighting, handrails and extra safety and security devices
- having common dining areas and providing meals—some included in the general fees paid, others charged extra—specially prepared for older tastes and digestion
- providing some laundry and housekeeping services, although there may be extra charges for these
- offering some commercial services on the premises, such as banking, a beauty salon, shops, a library, local transportation
- organizing social, educational and recreational events both on and off the premises, and

■ having a nurse or paramedic on duty, or other medical emergency system.

INDEPENDENT LIVING PLUS HOME CARE

You may be one of many people considering a move to an independent living community, but not certain that you are independent enough. You may need some of the personal care offered by assisted living, but not all of it. The difference may be something as simple as needing help to take a shower. And if you need only a little personal care, you may not want the close monitoring and regulations of assisted living, nor do you want to pay the higher cost for help you don't need. But without a small amount of extra care, you cannot quite manage on your own.

One solution may be for you to arrange for outside home care in your independent living residence. (See Chapter 2.) You may be able to hire just as much home care as you need, without the unwanted and costly care provided by assisted living. Some independent living facilities even maintain a roster of reliable outside home care providers and will help arrange the care.

Other independent living communities, however, have rules about the type or frequency of outside care permitted. And some independent living facilities require that all residents maintain a certain level of physical capability—being ambulatory and able to get in and out of bed unassisted, for example. Such rules may make home care in those communities less useful than it could be. (See Section A3.)

---

2. Costs

Independent living residences range from federally subsidized studio apartments rented for a few hundred dollars a month to luxury homes sold for over a million dollars. And there are other important questions to factor in about cost: Are there fees in addition to rent or purchase price? How much are rent and fees likely to be raised over time? What services are included in the price you pay and what services cost extra?

a. Renting

Many independent living complexes offer studio, one-bedroom or two-bedroom rental apartments. Because of the services, facilities, staff and common areas that are also provided, rent for these units generally runs 50% to 100% higher than for a comparable apartment in the same locale. On the other hand, they are usually 50% to 100% less expensive than comparable assisted living units. And a few seniors apartment buildings are federally subsidized, which means that the rents there are lower for those who meet the eligibility requirements of low fixed income and very few assets.

Although the initial rent for an independent living apartment may be affordable, you may also need to consider rent increases. Because they provide more than just housing, independent living complexes are almost always exempt from city or county rent control laws. However, you may be able to control your own rent for a short time through a lease. Most independent living facilities will offer a one-year lease; some will offer two or three years. Longer leases are rarely offered, and are probably not a good idea for you, either. If it turns out that you do not like living in the apartment, or your needs change and you can no longer manage in independent living, a long lease might tie you down.

Before moving into a rental apartment, ask to see the facility's record of rent increases over the previous five years. If it has consistently raised rents by large amounts, it is a good bet the practice will continue. On the other hand, if it has kept rent increases low over the years, it might also do so for the foreseeable future.

b. Buying

Many independent living complexes are enclosed subdivisions with single family homes or townhouses for sale. Also, many seniors apartments are sold as condominiums or cooperatives rather than rented. The prices of these houses and apartments vary widely, depending on size, quality, location and services. A seniors housing unit tends to have less square footage than regular housing with the same number of rooms, but their special design, security and included services make the properties more expensive.

Unlike open market housing, many seniors independent living complexes restrict an owner's rights to resell or mortgage the property. In all seniors housing, a new buyer must qualify under the community's general rules: be over a certain age and have a defined physical independence. (See Section A3.) But some complexes place additional restrictions on resale or refinance. For example, a housing complex may reserve the right to buy back the unit for some percentage more than the seller paid—or some percentage less than any offer the seller receives. And rules may also restrict an owner's right to refinance the house, or to obtain cash by taking out a reverse mortgage. (See Chapter 2, Section H.) There may also be strict rules against renting out the property.

If at some point you need to move to a higher level of care than you can receive in independent living, or for any other reason you want to move out, these restrictions may make it difficult to sell your home. They will also reduce its market value. Your survivors would experience the same difficulties if you died while living in the property. So, before entering into any agreement to purchase an independent living house or apartment, examine thoroughly any rules relating to resale or refinance. If you are not certain how those rules might affect you, get a full explanation from an attorney, accountant or other financial advisor who is not connected to the facility.

c. Additional fees

At many senior residences, the price or rent for a house or apartment is only one of several costs. There is often an entrance fee that is partially or entirely nonrefundable. Many residential complexes also charge monthly maintenance fees. And some places include certain services such as one daily meal and occasional cleaning services in the basic rent or purchase price, but charge extra fees for other services, such as additional meals, laundry and access to recreation.

Entrance fees. If you buy an independent living house or condominium, and in some cases if you rent, you may be required to pay a lump sum entrance fee, also called an endowment fee or a founders fee. These fees may range from $10,000 to $100,000—depending on how luxurious the place is, or how much in demand.

Sometimes, these entrance fees are fully refundable for a limited time; if you sell the unit within the first three to six months after you bought it, some housing complexes may refund the entire fee. At other places, you get back only a portion of the fee when you sell your unit; commonly, the entrance fee refund is reduced by 1% to 5% for each month you live in the residence.

Maintenance fees. Most independent living complexes in which the residents own their house or condominium charge a monthly maintenance fee. With rental units, the maintenance fees are usually part of the rent. There is a maintenance fee even if there was also an entrance fee. Before you buy a residence, find out if there are any rules that control how much the maintenance fee may be raised per year. If there are no rules about fee increases, check the facility's records for the previous five years to see how often and by how much the fees have been raised.

Fees for services. All independent living residences include some services in addition to a roof over your head. It is important to find out which services are included in the rent or purchase price plus maintenance fees, and which cost extra.

Most independent living residences have a kitchen and common dining room in which at least one hot meal per day is served; some serve three meals, although breakfast and lunch may be informal buffets. But meals may not be included in your regular rent or maintenance fees; if you want meals, you may have to pay extra for them. Food is usually a senior's greatest expense after rent and health care. Shopping for, preparing and cleaning up after meals can be a significant burden for many elders. And good nutrition is a key to continued good health. For all these reasons, finding out how many meals are included in your basic rent or maintenance fee, and how much extra meals cost, is an important part of your investigation of any independent living residence. Quality is important, too. If the residence's food will be something you count on, make sure to sample it; have at least two meals before you agree to move in.

INCLUSIVE CONTRACTS PROVIDE ALL THAT IS OFFERED

Some independent living complexes offer what is called an inclusive contract or extensive agreement, which means that the rent or purchase price plus maintenance fees include all the services the facility provides. If there is both an inclusive and a non-inclusive contract, you must determine if the extra cost of the inclusive contract is worth the extra services. If the extra services are not things you particularly care about, you may not want to pay for them.

The choice between the two types of contract is less difficult if you are permitted to pay for individual services without having to buy the whole inclusive package. Then you may be able to pick and choose the few extra services you want—lunch and sessions with an exercise instructor, for example—without having to pay for all the other things in the inclusive contract in which you're not as interested.

Among other services commonly offered are recreation—exercise and dance, for example, and golf, tennis and swimming at the more expensive communities. You may be charged a separate fee for some of these services, or charged extra for unlimited or preferential access to them. Similarly, transportation, housekeeping, laundry and shopping services may be offered, but some or all of them only for extra fees.

Another important service provided by some independent living facilities is temporary personal assistance. If you need long-term help with dressing, bathing, eating, or moving around, you will not be permitted to remain in independent living. (See Section A3.) But if your need for care is only short-term, some facilities provide it. Whether this kind of personal care is offered by a facility, and whether it is included in your regular fees or you must pay extra for it, is also important to determine before you sign up.

3. Rules and Restrictions

Because they are organized facilities rather than merely a collection of residences, independent living communities tend to have numerous rules and regulations by which residents must abide. The rules range from simple things like the time meals are served, or the decorations or modifications permitted in an individual living unit, to the extremely important matter of the physical condition a resident must maintain to live there.

a. Age and physical condition

Independent living facilities require that residents maintain a certain level of physical independence. There are usually two different standards: one to enter as a resident, another somewhat less stringent standard to remain.

Requirements to enter. To qualify to buy or rent a housing unit, you must have reached at least a minimum age—usually 55 or 60. But in many residence complexes you also may not be too old; some have entry limits of age 75, 80 or 85.

In most residences, you must also be fully ambulatory—meaning that you are able to move around without a wheelchair or personal assistance. Most independent living complexes permit a new resident to use a walker, but some do not permit the walkers or oxygen units in the common dining areas. Many independent living facilities also require that new residents be fully continent; others insist that a resident must not require assistance eating, at least in the common dining area.

Requirements to remain. Residents in independent living units might not be permitted to remain if their physical conditions deteriorate, for more than a short time, past a certain point. That point usually involves one or more of the following:

- inability to get in and out of bed without assistance
- full incontinence, or
- inability to eat without assistance.

Because of such rules, if you are already frail and are likely, within the foreseeable future, to fall below a residence's physical condition requirements, you should consider one of the following:

- an independent living residence with less stringent requirements, or with no requirements at all for continuing residents
- an assisted living residence instead of independent living (see Section B), or
- a facility with more than one level of care, so that if you must move, you will be able to remain in the same residential community. (See Section C.)

RULES FOR COUPLES

It often happens that one person in a couple—either a married couple, siblings or other combination of people who live together—loses some physical capabilities before the other does. If one of the couple falls below the facility's physical requirements to remain, yet the other remains physically qualified, what happens depends on the rules of the facility and the availability of another housing unit within the same complex.

In some residences, the couple must move—or one of them must move while the other remains. If the same facility offers assisted living units, this rule would not create quite as much of a hardship. Other facilities permit the couple to stay if the less able one can reach the minimum physical standards with the help of the healthier one, but without outside assistance.

Any couple considering an independent living residence must understand these rules, and make sure they are clearly spelled out in the written residence contract.

---

b. Number of residents, guests, assistants

Many independent living facilities limit the number of people who may live in any given unit. The maximum is usually two; only one might be permitted for small units. All residents must be over a certain age—generally 55 to 65. That means that children or grandchildren may not move in, even if they could provide needed personal care for the resident. Some communities also require that couples who share a residence be related. This restriction eliminates the great cost savings of sharing with a housemate—and it prohibits older couples who are not married.

Most residences also have rules regarding overnight guests. Some prohibit guests in the units but offer guest rooms or apartments for short stays, usually with an extra charge to the resident. Some permit guests for short stays, but prohibit children under a certain age. Most places allow guests for meals—charging extra to the resident; some even provide a separate, private dining room for groups or special occasions.

An important matter to investigate when you consider an independent living residence is whether and under what circumstances it permits home care for individual residents. Having a personal care aide come to your home on a regular basis to help you with activities of daily living—dressing, bathing, cooking and eating, getting in and out of bed, taking a walk—may mean the difference between remaining in independent living and having to move to assisted living or a nursing facility. But some residences limit the number of regular visits by outside personal care aides, or do not permit them at all except on a temporary basis while a resident recovers from an illness or injury. Such a restriction may not seem that meaningful to you if you are now hale and hardy, but it could become important if and when your physical condition takes a turn for the worse.

A CHANGE IN OWNERSHIP MAY NOT BE GOOD NEWS

Like many other businesses these days, seniors residences are frequently the target of takeovers by larger companies. National corporations that run seniors residences around the country are gobbling up good, low-cost, locally owned facilities. And when the ownership changes, the quality and the cost often change, too.

New owners often change things to make their acquisition more profitable, which may mean less comfort and higher costs for the residents. So, if you are considering moving into an independent or assisted living residence complex, find out how long the current owners have operated it. If it has been sold within the previous two years, talk with the staff and residents about recent changes.

Cuts in services and staff may be making residents less comfortable than they have been, and future cuts may make things worse. Also, you can no longer rely on what the previous owners did regarding rent or fee increases. Ask management for information on increases the new ownership has imposed not only at this residence but also at other facilities they operate, particularly ones they have recently purchased.

B. Assisted Living

Assisted living combines much of the homelike atmosphere of independent living with some of the personal care of a nursing facility. It provides extensive personal assistance and services, plus round-the-clock monitoring, that are not offered by independent living residences and that would be extremely expensive if arranged through home care. On the other hand, assisted living permits residents to maintain some of the privacy and independence that are lost in more institutional, and more expensive, nursing facilities. Assisted living is the fastest growing type of seniors residence—fitting the needs of millions of seniors who cannot make it entirely on their own, but who do not need nursing care.

The residences discussed in this section come under a variety of names: assisted living, sheltered care, residential care, board and care, boarding home, catered living, congregate living and group home. Although each facility or residence differs somewhat in the type of housing and level of services and staffing provided, all of them, regardless of name, have certain things in common. They provide:

- domestic services, including meals and housekeeping
- assistance with personal care and the activities of daily living (see Section 1b), but not nursing care, and
- close monitoring to help ensure residents' health and safety.

1. The Basics

Assisted living provides a room or small apartment—usually rented—intended to help maintain a homelike setting, plus a range of services to assist residents with those tasks of daily life made difficult for them by the loss of some physical or mental capabilities.

a. Types of living spaces

There are several kinds and sizes of assisted living housing: full-size one-bedroom apartments; studio apartments with small kitchenettes; studios without a kitchen, or with a partial kitchen that has no cooking facilities; single rooms; and shared rooms. An assisted living apartment or room may be furnished or unfurnished. Even if a space is furnished, at some places residents are permitted to bring in some furnishings of their own, which can make a new place feel more like home.

Assisted living apartments and rooms tend to be smaller than living spaces intended for the general public. They are often fitted with safety devices such as handrails and special bathroom fixtures, and may include a hospital bed if needed. In addition to the small rooms and space-eating fixtures, people tend to bring more of their own furnishings than would otherwise fit easily into the space. As a result, many assisted living apartments feel crowded and even smaller than they are. It is often difficult for a new resident to adjust to the smaller, more cramped quarters.

SPECIAL CARE FOR ALZHEIMER'S OR DISORIENTATION

Many people suffer mild symptoms from the early stages of Alzheimer's or other age-related disorientation. Their need for monitoring and assistance make independent living too difficult or dangerous, but they do not need the high level of care provided by a nursing facility. For them, assisted living is often an excellent solution.

However, the kind of assistance these people need is different from that required by those who have only physical limitations. The same assisted living residence that provides good care for someone with only physical frailties does not necessarily work well for a person with mild dementia. Most assisted living facility administrators will tell you that they are experienced with Alzheimer's residents. But it is the quality of that experience that counts. Most important is whether the staff is trained to handle the difficulties of dementia sufferers. You want staff trained to provide special attention to residents who are mildly disoriented—not merely to shuttle them from one place or activity to another, but if necessary to explain what is going on, without treating the residents as children.

If you are considering an assisted living facility for someone with mild disorientation problems, watch how the staff interacts with current residents who have similar difficulties. And pay close attention to how the staff—not just the administrator who gives you a tour—interacts with you or your loved one during a meal, an activity, or an explanation of facility rules.

b. Services provided

The main difference between assisted living and independent living residences (see Section A) is that assisted living meets a higher level of daily needs. While assisted living does not offer either the medical care or the level of attention of a nursing facility, it does provide personal care in a resident's living space as well as common areas, meals and household tasks, and extensive monitoring of each resident's physical condition.

Personal assistance. The reason most people move to assisted living is that they need help with one or more of what are known as the Activities of Daily Living (ADLs). ADLs include eating, bathing, dressing, continence and using the toilet, walking and getting in and out of bed or chair.

An assisted living facility will help a resident with any ADL, but not all the time, and not anytime a resident wants help. Instead, a schedule will be developed which takes into account the resident's needs and the staff's availability. For example, an aide might help a resident get in and out of bed in the morning, once or twice during the day, at bedtime and once again during the night. Or a resident will be given a full bath three or four times a week, but not every day.

When you consider a particular assisted living residence, ask precisely what it offers regarding the specific ADLs with which you need assistance. If the facility offers you the kind and frequency of assistance you believe fits your needs, make certain that care is spelled out in the written residence agreement you and the management sign.

Health monitoring. In addition to help with daily activities, assisted living facilities monitor a resident's health. That does not mean nursing or other active treatment of a medical condition. Rather, it means keeping track of and helping the resident take the correct dose of medications, helping the resident with self-administered health aids such as prostheses and oxygen, providing emergency call systems and checking on a resident's well-being during the night.

Most assisted living residences have a nurse on duty to check on any resident who has health difficulty, or whose physical condition seems to be changing, and to refer the resident for medical care if it seems necessary. Health monitoring may also include coordinating care with the resident's primary care physician and keeping track of a resident's medical appointments. And most facilities provide or arrange transportation to and from those appointments.

STRICT RULES ARE A PROBLEM FOR SOME PEOPLE

Assisted living offers close monitoring of residents' physical conditions. This includes keeping track of medications, checking on residents at night and making sure residents eat properly. Assisted living facilities accomplish this by setting up schedules and requiring both staff and residents to follow them.

Sometimes, these schedules and rules are too restrictive for a competent, independent-minded person. (See Section B3, below.)

Depending on your needs, including your need to be left alone, independent living plus home care might fit your personality better than assisted living—even though that arrangement places the burden on you and your family to organize care.

Meals. One of the most attractive things for many people about assisted living is that meals are provided. There is a kitchen and a common dining room where at least two and usually three meals a day are served, and their costs are part of the resident's rent or fees. Residents are freed from shopping, cooking and cleaning up; they are assured of nutritious food; and they are brought together for the informal social exchange of a meal with other residents.

There are several things to check about an assisted living residence's food service. First is how many meals a day are included, and whether they are all full, hot meals. Then there is the quality of the food; it won't do you any good if you won't eat it. Try several meals in their dining room, and see if the residents seem interested in their food and in each other.

It is also important to find out what happens if a resident is not able to appear for a meal, or simply does not want a meal in the dining room. Are meals served at different times, or only at one set time? Under what circumstances are meals delivered to individual rooms or apartments? May a resident take food from the dining room back to a private room? If three meals a day are served, may a resident regularly choose not to appear for one or more of them? If so, does the resident need to prove to the staff that he or she is getting enough nutrition without the prepared meal?

Housekeeping. Assisted living facilities provide laundry service and also clean individual rooms or apartments. What that housekeeping includes, however, can vary considerably. How often are a resident's bedding and bath linen laundered? Does the facility do a resident's personal laundry as well? Is there an extra charge for personal laundry? How often is an individual room or apartment cleaned?

Social activities and exercise. It is one thing to assist residents with the basics of daily life such as dressing and bathing; that help is guaranteed in a contract with an assisted living residence. It may be quite another thing to help residents to lead mentally, physically and socially active lives. This is not a matter of contract, but of the fabric of service at a good residence. Most facilities plan group activities such as guest lectures and exercise classes, as well as regular gatherings for the residents to visit among themselves. The best facilities also help individual residents participate in these activities to the extent possible, and provide alternatives—an assisted walk around the hallways, for example, or a one-on-one chat in a resident's private room—when it's not feasible to participate in a group.

There are several ways to get a sense of the quality of group and individual activities at a particular facility. You can take a look at what is scheduled for any given week, but it is also important to visit during one of these planned activities to see if residents participate and seem to enjoy doing so. As for more individual attention, find out whether there are any rules against staff spending non-scheduled time with residents. And on all your visits, watch how the staff interact with residents: look for a friendly, relaxed manner on both parts. (See Chapter 4, Section B, for information on how to choose a nursing facility, much of which also applies to assisted living.)

2. Costs

Most assisted living spaces are rented, not purchased. The major exception is assisted living as part of a continuing care community. (See Section C2.)

a. Basic rent

Obviously, rent depends on the size of living space. A small room with no cooking facilities is much less than a spacious one-bedroom apartment with full kitchen. The rent also varies with the amount of services and staff provided, the location and the overall condition of the facility. And some facilities offer more than one type of rental agreement: a limited contract may include fewer meals and personal assistance than an inclusive or extensive agreement that includes all the services the facility has to offer. Given all these variables, rent for an assisted living unit generally runs 50% to 100% higher than for a comparable independent living unit in the same facility. But they are still one-third to one-half the cost of nursing facilities of the same quality, in the same area.

b. Rent increases

As with any other rental housing, you must consider how much your rent may go up over time. A lease can guarantee the rent for a year or two. After that, rent increases are completely up to the facility's ownership, unless a yearly limit is included in your rental agreement. Without such a limit, it is important to check a facility's record of rent increases over the previous five years. If they have raised rents in large chunks, you have to consider whether they will price you out of your apartment in years to come.

c. Additional fees

Some assisted living facilities charge fees in addition to rent. There may be a one-time non-refundable entrance fee. And there may be a fee for certain services not included in the basic assisted living contract: extra or delivered meals; extra housekeeping service; local transportation fees; personal care beyond the standard level of care offered in the facility.

d. Medicaid coverage

Medicaid (called Medi-Cal in California) is a federal program, administered somewhat differently by each state, that pays medical expenses for people with very low incomes and few assets. (See Chapter 6.)

Until very recently, Medicaid has paid for home care and for nursing facility care, but not for any type of long-term care residence in between. Slowly, however, Medicaid administrators have begun to recognize that many people who live in nursing facilities paid for by Medicaid could be living more comfortably in much less expensive assisted living facilities if only Medicaid would pay for it. So, a number of states are now exploring the advantages of paying for assisted living for some people who would otherwise qualify for nursing facility care.

These programs are just getting underway, however, and there are no national standards that establish when and where Medicaid will pay for assisted living. Medicaid assisted living coverage is currently available in only a few states, sometimes only in certain counties, and usually on a temporary, experimental basis. Also, even where the program exists, most assisted living residences are not certified to accept Medicaid.

Nonetheless, if you believe you might qualify for Medicaid now, or might qualify in the foreseeable future after spending most of your assets, it would be wise to take a number of steps.

- Read Chapter 6 of this book regarding Medicaid eligibility.
- Contact the Medicaid office in the county in which you are looking at assisted living residences to find out if the local program covers assisted living and if so, what the rules are.
- If Medicaid does cover some assisted living, get a list from the Medicaid office of all the assisted living facilities in the area that are certified to receive Medicaid payments.

Note that it may be better to get the information about whether a particular facility is covered directly from a Medicaid office rather than from facility administrators. If the facility does not accept Medicaid, your question may scare off the facility operators even if you are currently able to pay your own way. They might worry that you are asking about Medicaid because you will not have the money to pay for very long, and so might not want to take you on as a resident.

e. Long-term care insurance coverage

Virtually none of the private long-term care insurance policies issued during the 1970s and 1980s covers assisted living: they are all essentially nursing home policies, some of which also cover home care. By the mid-1990s, however, some policies began to offer coverage for assisted living. This was due in part to increased competition among insurance companies, and in part to the insurance companies' realization that if they have to pay on a policy, they would rather pay for assisted living than for a more expensive nursing facility.

If you have long-term care insurance and believe assisted living might be a better choice for you than either home care or a nursing facility, check the extent of coverage in your policy. If assisted living is covered, carefully examine the requirements to qualify under your particular policy.

In general, such policies require that you must have physical or mental limitations that trigger the coverage: usually the need for assistance with at least two or three Activities of Daily Living, or ADLs. (See Section B1.) Some policies make this requirement a bit easier to meet by also looking at what are called instrumental ADLs; these include the abilities to keep house, to manage money and bills and to manage medications.

There is also the question of who decides whether your condition meets these standards. The policy may require that your primary care physician certify that you meet the conditions, but the policy may also permit the insurance company to have its own doctor examine you before agreeing that the coverage trigger has been met. (See Chapter 10.)

3. Rules and Restrictions

Assisted living facilities take on the difficult task of providing different types and amounts of care and services to people who, like everyone else, have individual quirks and personality traits. One way these facilities manage this is to set standards regarding who is an appropriate resident, and to create fairly strict rules by which all residents must abide.

a. Becoming and remaining a resident

Just as assisted living fits between independent living and nursing care, its residents' physical and mental capabilities are supposed to fit between complete independence and total dependence. To ensure this fit, assisted living facilities establish standards for residents to enter and to remain.

The entrance testing for potential residents may begin with a minimum age—55 or 60—and sometimes a maximum—80 or 85. Then there is the matter of the care needed by a potential resident. Facilities will usually accommodate a person with little need for assistance who wants the personal attention offered by an assisted living facility and is willing to pay for it; some facilities with few vacancies, however, might suggest that a relatively healthy potential resident try independent living instead. But assisted living facilities are usually careful not to accept a resident who needs more care than they can deliver. So most of them scrupulously assess each potential resident's physical and cognitive capabilities before agreeing to let the individual into the facility.

Rules for entering and staying in such facilities commonly mandate that residents:

- require regular staff assistance with no more than two to four of the Activities of Daily Living (ADLs)—eating, bathing, dressing, transferring in and out of bed and chair, using the toilet, walking
- not be completely incontinent
- not require daily nursing care, and
- not present a danger to themselves, staff or other residents and do not require extremely close monitoring or physical control—unless the facility has a special care unit for Alzheimer's or other dementia sufferers.

Unless it is part of a continuing care community in which each resident is guaranteed the right to remain in whatever level of care is required (see Section C2), an assisted living facility may force a resident to move out—usually to a nursing facility—if he or she falls below the facility's standards of physical or mental condition.

However, assisted living facilities are often more flexible with existing residents than with potential ones. For example, a facility may permit a resident to remain if he or she hires outside assistance for the extra care the facility is unable to provide. That, in turn, may depend on other facility rules regarding how much outside assistance is permitted.

WHO DECIDES WHETHER YOU MUST MOVE?

A resident must meet physical standards to remain in an assisted living facility. But who decides exactly what a resident's condition is? Since the most likely alternative is having to move to a nursing facility, the question may prove to be an extremely important one.

Some things are obvious. If a resident becomes completely bedridden, there is no argument that he or she still meets the facility's standards. But often, the issue is murky. The degree of a resident's incontinence may be unclear, for example. Or a disabling condition might be permanent, but the resident might also slowly recover from it.

An assisted living contract should clearly describe how this decision is made. Facilities always reserve the right to make the final decision. But the decision should also take into account the resident's primary care physician's opinion and should also be reviewed by an independent physician or geriatric social worker.

---

b. Outside assistance

Some assisted living residences place strict limits on visits by outside nurses and personal care aides. Some permit them only on a temporary basis while a resident recovers from an illness or injury. Others permit regular visits by outside help, but limit the type or frequency. If the personal care assistance offered by an assisted living facility does not seem to match your needs, but you believe you can fill the gaps with outside help, find out whether the facility's rules would permit it. If so, make sure the rules are clearly spelled out in your written residence agreement.

c. Staff control over residents

One of the important services provided by assisted living staff is round-the-clock monitoring of the residents' well-being. Part of this is often achieved through strict schedules by which staff and residents must abide. For example, meals might be served at a precise hour, and residents must appear in the dining room for all of them. Or a staff aide might enter each resident's room one or more times every night to check on the resident's condition. Or the staff might control all of a resident's medications, even non-prescription ones, to ensure proper and timely use and to protect against adverse drug interactions.

For some residents, however, this constant caretaking is more than they need or want. It is therefore important to find out not only the facility's rules and schedules but also its flexibility. For example, if a resident does not want three meals a day in the dining room, do the rules allow checking in without having to appear? Can some meals be delivered to a resident's quarters or must the resident provide his or her own food if a meal is skipped? Can nightly check-ups be eliminated if the resident finds them more disturbing than beneficial? May medications be left with the resident if the resident has sufficient awareness and orientation to monitor them without help?

d. Right to return after an absence

Many assisted living residents have serious medical crises that force them into the hospital and a nursing or rehabilitation center for extended stays. Often no one knows for months whether the resident will recover sufficiently to again live in assisted living, or instead will need to move to a long-term care nursing facility. During these months, the resident may not want or be able to pay for an assisted living room or apartment that is not being used and to which the resident might not return.

Most facilities have rules regarding a resident's right to return after an extended absence. Many facilities will hold a room or apartment for a short time, then offer a longer period—often six months or a year—during which the former resident has priority over new applicants for the next available equivalent room or apartment. Without such protection in an assisted living contract, one serious medical crisis could mean that, even if you eventually recover, you would have to search for a new home.

C. Combination Residential Facilities

The first two sections of this chapter discuss independent living communities and assisted living residences, while Chapter 4 covers nursing facilities. But many senior communities combine two or three of these levels in one place. This section explains the different combinations, their benefits and risks.

1. Multi-Level Residences

Many seniors residence communities offer both independent living and assisted living in the same complex of buildings and grounds. Because many design features and services are common to both, it can be economical for the same ownership to build and operate the two levels together. This makes it possible for a senior to move into an independent living residence and conveniently transfer to assisted living if necessary.

The fact that both independent living and assisted living are offered within the same seniors community, however, does not necessarily mean that you may move from one to the other whenever you choose. In a multi-level community, you may be given the opportunity to move from one level to another, but not a guarantee. This differentiates it from continuing care and life care communities in which, for considerably more money than a simple multi-level facility, you lock in the right to move to a different level as needed. (See Section C2.)

In a multi-level community, an independent living resident may move to assisted living only if there is a vacant unit that fits the resident's needs and budget. Some people move into assisted living first, and then to independent living if they regain strength or mobility. But most move first into independent living and later to assisted living.

If there is no vacancy when needed, the resident must wait. This is not always a major problem, since the need for more care often develops slowly, as a person's physical strength diminishes. And the wait may be shorter if the facility gives priority for vacancies to existing residents. That should be spelled out in the written residency agreement.

If you do eventually need assisted living, a multi-level community offers advantages that may make it worth the potential delay.

- You can remain within a familiar physical setting and routine. In most places, many of the community's common areas are used by both independent living and assisted living. And although your private living space would change when you move from one level to another, it would still have a familiar look and feel—in design, bath and kitchen fixtures, for example.

- Many of the people on staff will be the same, so you don't need to get to know a whole new crew, and they don't need to become newly acquainted with you.

- The other residents whom you have come to know will still be your neighbors.

- You avoid the strenuous and always disorienting process of packing up, moving to a new location, settling in and getting to know a new area, a new living space, new rules and regulations, new people.

2. Continuing Care Retirement Communities (CCRCs)

A Continuing Care Retirement Community (CCRC) provides any level of care and services you need—independent living, assisted living or custodial nursing care—for as long as you are a resident. (See Chapter 4 for information on custodial level nursing care.) The basic agreement of a CCRC is that the resident pays a hefty entry fee and monthly charges to live in the community, and the facility guarantees that the resident may move from one level of care to another as the resident's physical and mental condition require. The phrase often used to describe this guarantee is "aging in place"—that is, to live in the same place through all the stages of growing old. And while some CCRCs truly offer an "age in place" guarantee, others fudge a bit on the "place." (See Section 2a.)

Some CCRCs offer a year-to-year arrangement to residents, after an initial entrance fee. These facilities may also have monthly maintenance fees; these fees are sometimes tiered—meaning that they are higher for assisted living than for independent living, and highest for nursing care. Other CCRCs offer an extended lease, which locks in maintenance fees and other charges for the period of the lease. And a special, extra expensive kind of CCRC arrangement, called a Life Care contract, promises care for as long as the resident lives. (See Section 2d.)

a. Basic arrangements

All CCRCs provide continuing care, but not all of them do so in the same location. Almost all CCRCs offer independent living and assisted living in the same place. And some CCRCs also have an onsite nursing facility. But many CCRCs have no separate nursing wing; instead, a resident who needs nursing care must receive it in an assisted living apartment, and when that is not practical, must move into a separate offsite nursing facility with which the CCRC has a contractual arrangement.

ONSITE OR OFFSITE NURSING FACILITIES

A CCRC with its own nursing facility is not necessarily better than one that has contracted with an outside facility. In fact, some onsite nursing facilities are no more than rooms in a separate section of assisted living where nursing care is delivered. Of course, there are advantages to remaining in the same location with some of the same staff and your neighbors nearby. But if an onsite nursing wing does not get much of the community's attention, expertise and money, it may be better to move to an offsite nursing facility that provides only one level of care and does it well.

Find out whether a CCRC's onsite nursing facility is certified by the state. If not, find out whether it contracts with a separate local nursing facility to take residents for whom they can no longer care. If it does, visit that facility and assess it as thoroughly as possible. (See Chapter 4.)

Beware that some CCRCs only admit residents who are initially able to qualify for independent living. That is because it costs less for the CCRC to provide care and services for an independent living resident, and the facility administrators want to make sure that they get several years of providing this less expensive level of service before they have to provide more costly assisted living or nursing care. Some CCRCs also have a maximum entry age of around 80.

LOOK CLOSELY AT DISTANT OBJECTS

People who consider moving into a CCRC do so because they want to provide not only for their immediate needs, but also for those down the road. Unfortunately, when investigating specific communities, too many people focus on the independent living quarters and services where they would first live, and only casually look into the assisted living and nursing facility care. This nearsightedness is often encouraged by the community's sales staff, who know that independent living is always a more cheerful and inviting part of the community to show a prospective resident.

Investigate the assisted living and nursing facility living quarters, services and costs as closely as you do independent living. You may never need those levels of care, but if you do, you will want them to measure up. You will have already paid a lot of money for them. And if someday you need the care they offer, you will have to depend on them. This advice is important for all CCRCs, but doubly so if you are considering a Life Care contract. (See Section 2d.)

---

b. Costs

Because of its guarantee of care and services at any level needed at any time, a house or apartment in a CCRC is usually substantially more expensive than a comparable living space in a multi-unit facility that offers no nursing care and that provides no transfer guarantee.

Rentals. If an independent living house or apartment in a CCRC is offered as a rental, you can expect to pay anywhere from 25% to 100% more than a comparable rental in a non-CCRC independent living community. The amount of rent may depend on how steep the entry and maintenance fees are; sometimes high fees mean lower rent.

The rent may also depend on the level of care and services you receive. That is, while you have guaranteed access to assisted living or nursing care if you need it, there may be higher rent for those levels than for independent living.

A potential resident must also look into the possibility of rent increases. Some facilities agree in the rental contract to a percentage limit on rent increases. Others have no such limit, however. If there is no contractual limit on rent increases, it is important to investigate the facility's recent record on that score. (See Section A2.)

Purchases. Some CCRCs offer equity purchases rather than rentals. This usually means that you are buying an interest in a specific condominium. But in other CCRCs, you buy an interest in the whole community—a membership, so to speak—which does not give you ownership, and the right to sell, any particular living unit.

How resale works—what you have to sell and under what terms—is a crucial aspect of a CCRC agreement. If you buy into a CCRC, you must fully understand the limits placed on your ability to resell your interest if someday you choose to move out, as well as the equity that may remain for your survivors if you die while still living in the community. (See Section A2.)

Entrance and maintenance fees. There is usually a large entrance fee that is only partially refundable, and only for a short time, should you decide to move out of the CCRC. Fees range from $50,000 to $300,000 and up. In addition to the overall quality of and demand for space in the particular CCRC, the entrance fee may vary with the size of the independent living unit and the type of nursing care contract.

There may also be monthly maintenance fees. Those fees may increase if you move from one level to another. And the amounts will go up over time. In the best residence contracts, the percentage that maintenance may be raised per year is strictly limited. If it is not limited at all, fee increases over the years could eat up your savings and, if you could no longer afford them, force you to move out.

Nursing care fees. Although all CCRCs guarantee nursing care should it become necessary, the terms of that care vary greatly from one community to another. Whether the care is provided onsite or in a separate facility was discussed above. (See Section C2.) But there is also the question of extra charges for nursing care, depending on where and for how long you receive it. Different types of residence contracts cover these variables in nursing care fees. Some communities offer only one type of contract; others offer a choice, at different prices.

- An extensive or all-inclusive CCRC contract provides unlimited nursing facility care of all levels, either onsite or in a separate facility, without any extra charge. (See Chapter 4.) Because there is no limit to how much expensive nursing care you might receive under such terms, the entrance and monthly fees for these contracts are the highest. A Life Care contract includes unlimited nursing care. (See Section C2.)

- A modified CCRC contract guarantees a certain number of days per year of free nursing care—usually 30 to 90 days. The number of days may vary depending on whether the care is delivered onsite or requires moving to a separate nursing facility. After the free days have been used, you are charged additional fees, which may range from $25 to $200 per day, depending on the level of care provided. These contracts are less expensive than all-inclusive arrangements.

- A fee-for-service CCRC contract guarantees you nursing care as needed, provided in your living unit, in the community's own nursing wing, or in a specific separate facility, but charges you a daily fee for the care. The amount of the fee often varies, depending on the level of nursing care you receive and where you receive it. Because these charges partially offset the community's cost of providing nursing care, the entrance and monthly fees for such a contract are the lowest.

c. Decisions about levels of care

It is one thing to know that many levels of services and care are available to you in a CCRC. It is another thing to know who decides which level of care is needed. No CCRC permits a resident to have the sole authority to decide what level of care is appropriate. On the other hand, you should not enter any CCRC that reserves for itself the exclusive right to decide when to move you in or out of independent living, assisted living or nursing care.

A CCRC should have specific written standards, made part of the residence contract, that spell out what physical or mental conditions require or permit residence in one community level or another. Whether you need nursing care should be determined by your primary care physician. The CCRC, however, may reserve the right to decide whether you are to receive that nursing care in your residence, in a nursing care wing of the community, or in a separate, offsite nursing facility. That decision should be made only after the community's management obtains an assessment of your condition and needs from a physician, nursing supervisor or geriatric social worker, in consultation with your primary care physician.

d. Life Care contracts

One form of arrangement with a CCRC provides care for the life of the resident. A Life Care contract makes a very large promise: If you enter a residence in your 70s, as many people do, the facility might have to provide you with 20 or 30 years of care. In exchange, the entrance fee is extremely high—$100,00 to $500,000, or more. And that may not include the cost of your individual residence and other fees. In other words, that may be merely the cost of your lifetime membership in the community.

Because your investment is so large, you must judge a Life Care contract and the community that offers it with extraordinary care.

What you buy with a Life Care contract is no different from what you get in any other CCRC; it is just guaranteed to last longer. And the length of the contract is the source of its two major potential problems. First is uncertainty concerning the quality of care the community will provide in the future. The other is the amount of monthly maintenance charges the facility will levy years down the road.

A resident is not handcuffed to the community. If the quality of care and services becomes poor, or the maintenance fees too high, you are free to leave. But you will have lost the lifetime benefit your huge entrance fee was intended to cover. And losing that money may make a move somewhere else unaffordable. Also, if you have purchased an equity interest in specific living quarters, the contract terms may prevent you from recouping much of your equity when you sell.

Diminished quality. There are many scenarios in which a dazzlingly luxurious and well-staffed Life Care community becomes unable to provide high-quality services after 10, 20 or more years. The operators of the community may not have calculated fees and costs properly, or may be poor administrators and squander the funds needed to maintain high-quality premises, services and care over the long haul. Or the buildings and equipment may not be constructed to last, and may require unaffordable refurbishing. And there is the problem of profit-taking: Owners may take out of the business too much money for themselves, leaving too little to maintain high-quality operations. Similarly, the business may be sold, with new operators committed more to their profits than to the quality of care.

Increased fees. Either to make up for poor planning and management, or simply to increase profits, the owners might begin to raise monthly maintenance and nursing care surcharges at a steeper rate as both you and the facility age. Unless your contract has narrow limits regarding how much the fees and surcharges may be raised, they may get to levels that are difficult for you to pay, or that eat up the money you had intended to pass on to your survivors or to use for other purposes.

PREVENTION IS THE ONLY CURE

Because of the enormity of the investment and the many ways in which that investment may be at risk for the long term, you should thoroughly understand the terms of any Life Care contract and the financial condition of the facility and its owners. Before you enter into a Life Care contract, it is important to have a financial advisor, lawyer or accountant review all documents, investigate the financial status and reputation of the facility and its ownership and carefully explain to you the implications of that information.

Among the things an adviser should discuss with you are:

- **Terms of resale.** Do you own an equity interest in a specific piece of property or only a membership in the community? What are the terms under which your ownership interest may be sold, if at all, or left to your survivors?
- **Refund of entrance fee.** What amount of your entrance fee may be refunded to you if you decide to move out of the community?
- **Fee increases.** What are the limits on increases of monthly maintenance fees for each level of care, and on surcharges for nursing care?
- **Level of care.** Who decides the level of care and services you need, and how is that decision made?
- **Status of nursing facility.** Does the community maintain its own nursing facility onsite, and if so, is it certified by the state? If the community contracts with a separate offsite nursing facility, what are the terms of their agreement?
- **Financial stability.** Do the financial records of the facility indicate that it is on sound footing? What is the financial record and reputation of the parent company that owns the community? Are there any bankruptcies in the company's history? Is there a substantial reserve fund to cover unexpected decreases in revenues or increases in operating costs? ∎

Nursing Facilities

Despite a significant recent increase in home care and alternative seniors residences, nearly one out of every two women and one of four men over age 65 will enter a nursing facility some time in their lives. Many nursing facility stays are short ones while recuperating from an illness, injury or surgery. But many other stays are extended, expensive stays in a long-term care nursing facility: 25% of all nursing facility stays last more than a year and many last three years or more.

PLANNING AND FINANCES

If at all possible, thinking about and searching for a nursing facility should not be a hurried, emergency procedure. As soon as you begin to see that current living arrangements may become insufficient and neither home care nor assisted living will provide needed care or monitoring, begin planning.

Even finding out what nursing facility might be the best in a particular area can take time. And many good ones operate at full capacity and may not be able to accept a new resident at short notice.

You must also consider how a nursing facility will be paid. Family assets and income have to be calculated, along with reverse mortgages (see Chapter 2) and the amounts that might be contributed by Medicare and veterans' benefits (see Chapter 5) and any long-term care insurance (see Chapter 10). Medicaid coverage may be available for people with low income and few assets other than a home. (See Chapter 6.) It helps to understand Medicaid rules both to save some assets by advance planning and to recognize how much money might need to be repaid to Medicaid if the program pays for long-term nursing facility care.

There is a great range in the levels of care available in what are broadly termed "nursing facilities." Hospital-based skilled nursing facilities provide short-term, intensive medical care and monitoring for people recovering from acute illness or injury. Other facilities— what used to be called "rest homes"—provide long-term room and board and 24-hour assistance with personal care such as dressing, eating and moving about and daily nursing and other health care monitoring, though no intensive medical treatment.

Many people would prefer to remain outside a nursing facility but because of their condition, circumstances or the unavailability of in-home services or affordable assisted living residences, they can only receive adequate care in a residential nursing facility. Unfortunately, as sometimes makes the news, some facilities exist with substandard living conditions and even dangerous lack of care. Still others give basic care that meets technical health standards but offer little else, and have an atmosphere that is debilitating or demoralizing to the residents.

There are, however, excellent nursing facilities that provide high-quality care while assisting residents to maintain active lives with a full measure of dignity. But because there are many levels and types of nursing and personal care, the task is to find a good, affordable facility that is right for you.

WHERE TO FIND NURSING FACILITY REFERRALS

Hospital discharge planner. They will often be available for advice if you are going straight from a hospital to a nursing facility.

Your doctor. Ask your doctor about personal experience he or she may have had with area nursing facilities.

Organization focusing on specific illness. Check with organizations that focus on your particular illness or disability, such as the American Heart Association, American Cancer Society, American Diabetes Association, or Alzheimer's Disease Foundation.

National long-term care organizations. A number of private organizations such as American Association of Homes for the Aging specialize in long-term care and give referrals to local facilities. (See the Resource Directory in the Appendix.)

Government agencies. You can often get targeted referrals from the federal area Agencies on Aging, or from state and local agencies found through Senior Referral and Information numbers in the white pages of the phone book or your local county social services or family services agency.

Church, ethnic or fraternal organizations. Ask about nursing facilities members have used successfully or that are operated by or affiliated with the church or organization.

Relatives, friends and neighbors. They may have had experience with a nursing facility or know someone who has. They are often your best source of information.

A. Levels of Care

Care in nursing facilities ranges from intensive 24-hour care for the seriously ill, which is called skilled nursing care, to long-term personal assistance and health monitoring with very little active nursing, or custodial care. Some nursing facilities provide only one level of care, while others provide several levels at the same location.

Most people who are in nursing facilities cannot function without 24-hour monitoring and extensive personal assistance and nursing care because of illness or physical or mental limitations. But some residents are in relatively good physical and mental health, but too frail to live alone at home. If they had more family or resources, many of these people might be able to make do with extensive home care (see Chapter 2) or residence in an assisted living facility (see Chapter 3). For lack of an alternative, they become nursing facility residents.

In any case, the task is to find a good and affordable nursing facility that provides not just care, but the right type of care. For someone with severe physical or mental limitations, it is crucial to find a facility that provides the kind of attention and care that meets the individual's specific needs. For people who need little or no actual nursing care, the task is to find a facility that provides physical, mental and social stimulation rather than merely bed and food.

The hardest part may be footing the bill. Nursing facilities of all levels are very expensive, but depending on the type of care needed and the type of insurance you have, you may get some help covering the cost. Skilled nursing facilities run between $200 and $500 per day, although stays there are relatively short and Medicare or private health insurance usually pick up much of the tab. (See Chapter 5.) Custodial nursing facility care—the kind that may last for years— costs between $3,000 and $10,000 per month. Neither Medicare nor medi-gap private insurance supplements pay any of the cost of custodial care. Long-term care insurance, for those who have it, may cover some of the cost of custodial care. (See Chapter 10.) And Medicaid pays the full cost of custodial nursing facility care for people with very low income and few assets. (See Chapters 6 and 7.) Some veterans may also find coverage for custodial care through the Veterans Administration. (See Chapter 5.)

If a facility is certified by the federal government, it may also be more affordable. The Health Care Financing Administration has certified about 85% of all nursing facilities; HCFA certification means that the facility is eligible to receive Medicare and Medicaid payments. Some facilities do not meet HCFA standards. Other facilities charge high prices and simply do not want to accept residents who depend on Medicaid payments. Unless you have an unlimited supply of money to pay for long-term care, make sure that any facility you consider is certified. Certification means that the facility meets some certain minimum health, safety and care standards. And certification also means that if someday you should need and qualify for Medicaid coverage for your stay, you will be able to receive it without having to move to a different facility.

1. Hospital-Based Skilled Nursing Facilities

Hospital-based skilled nursing facilities, also known as extended care facilities, are departments within hospitals. They provide the highest levels of medical and nursing care, including 24-hour monitoring and intensive rehabilitative therapies. They are intended to follow acute hospital care due to serious illness, injury or surgery.

Unlike other nursing facilities, hospital-based facilities are not for permanent residence, but for a short term until a patient can be sent home or maintained elsewhere. Hospital-based facilities are very expensive ($200 to $500 per day), but the average stay is generally almost always for a matter of weeks only and, for those who qualify, is usually well covered by Medicare or private insurance. (See Chapters 5 and 10.)

2. Skilled Nursing Facilities

Non-hospital-based skilled nursing facilities (SNFs) provide a relatively high level of nursing and other medical care, as well as personal care and assistance, for people whose illnesses or impairments require close monitoring.

Around-the-clock nursing is available from licensed vocational or practical nurses, with at least one supervising registered nurse on duty at all times. In addition to nursing, most other prescribed medical services can be provided, including various rehabilitative therapies. A SNF is almost always for short-term recovery from a serious illness, injury or surgery that required hospitalization. A few people may spend months in a SNF, but most stays are for a matter of days or weeks.

The cost of SNF care ranges from $200 to $500 per day. Medicare, Medicaid and private insurance will pay for SNF care, but only up to specific coverage limits.

3. Intermediate Care Facilities

Intermediate care facilities (ICFs) provide less nursing and other medical care than SNFs. ICFs are for long-term residents with chronic illness or impairment whose conditions are not as acute as those of SNF residents and who are usually ambulatory.

Staff is geared as much toward personal care and assistance as to medical care, although there is always a licensed vocational or practical nurse on duty. ICFs generally care for people who need a long recovery period from serious illness, injury or surgery, but who no longer need quite the level of nursing care and high-tech monitoring that a SNF provides.

Costs range from $150 to $400 per day. There is no coverage by Medicare and private insurance coverage is rare, probably with prior approval required. Medicaid, however, may cover much of the cost of ICF care. (See Chapter 6.)

Very few facilities are set up to be ICFs alone; most are part of a SNF or a custodial care facility. (See Section 4.)

4. Custodial Care Facilities

The type of facility that houses long-term residents provides what is called custodial care: personal assistance and low-level nursing care, but not intensive medical care. Sometimes referred to as rest homes or nursing homes, these custodial care facilities (CCFs) are considerably less expensive than SNFs or ICFs and provide social and educational activities, as well as organized exercise, in addition to monitoring residents' physical conditions. Because CCFs do not provide extensive medical care, they are appropriate for people whose physical and mental conditions do not require constant attention or intervention.

Because of the limited medical and nursing care they offer, CCFs cost about $100 to $250 per day, considerably less than SNFs or ICFs. However, the length of stay in a CCF is often months or years at a cost of $35,000 to $100,000 per year. CCFs come in all shapes and sizes, from 20-bed facilities in converted private buildings with homey atmospheres to 100-bed facilities with large common areas and extensive social, physical and educational activities.

The remainder of this chapter discusses how to choose the facility that fits a particular individual's needs and budget.

5. Facilities for Alzheimer's or Dementia Sufferers

Many people who suffer from Alzheimer's or other forms of dementia need regular, close monitoring and considerable personal assistance.

They need the intense care provided by a nursing facility, but a different kind of care than is required by people who have only physical limitations. Not all facilities that provide good care for people with physical limitations do a good job with residents who suffer from dementia.

Some nursing facilities specialize in care for people with Alzheimer's or other disorientation. A few provide this type of care exclusively. More commonly, a general nursing facility will have a separate section or wing—often referred to as a Special Care or Dementia Unit.

To be effective and humane, the special care must consist of more than mere segregation from other residents. Some places are physically constructed to address the problems of disorientation: a circular design to ease traveling about; few doors, none unlocked to the outside; a protected interior courtyard or patio for fresh air and exercise; a plan and a place for nighttime wanderers; electronic or video monitoring. But most important, good facilities provide staff who are specially trained to handle the difficulties of dementia sufferers rather than relying on medications and restraints.

Unfortunately, the special unit or wing at some facilities offers little more than a higher price. The fact that a facility has a separate unit does not guarantee that the care provided there is particularly well suited to dementia sufferers. As with all the other aspects of a nursing facility, base your assessment of such a unit on the information you receive from your eyes and ears more than what you glean from brochures or sales pitches.

B. Choosing the Right Facility

Once you have determined which facilities in your area are affordable and provide the appropriate general level of care, you must decide which one best suits your needs and preferences.

The experts to turn to for guidance are the residents themselves. Most nursing facility residents, studies have shown, care very little about high-tech medical gear, or even about medical care. Rather, their most important concerns involve their ability to maintain some independence, to participate in decisions about daily life and to retain contact with the outside world.

Because so many of these and other concerns discussed below cannot be guaranteed in writing or demonstrated in a quick tour, it is important to spend as much time as possible at a facility before making a decision to receive care there. Make separate visits during the day, evening and night, and during one or more meals. And to the extent possible, talk with current residents and their families.

1. Ownership and Management

The quality of daily life in a nursing facility is determined primarily by on-site management and hands-on care personnel. And the owners of a nursing facility determine how well management can do its job through the funding provided for equipment, food and staffing. However, the form of ownership may not instruct about the quality of care any particular facility provides.

For-Profit Facilities

About three-fourths of all nursing facilities are operated for profit, many of them owned by big corporations. There is a popular but not necessarily accurate belief that in profit-making facilities, the dominating desire to make money means skimping on patient care. Research has shown that this is sometimes, but not always the case. Profit-making facilities may be better managed than nonprofit ones and therefore deliver better care for the dollar. Similarly, studies have found that keeping patients satisfied is important to for-profit facilities because their economic health depends on keeping their beds filled. As a result, a for-profit facility may be just as likely as a nonprofit facility to provide good quality care for the price.

Nonprofit Facilities

The flip-side of negative beliefs about profit-making facilities is the notion that those run by nonprofit philanthropic, charitable or religious organizations will provide quality care because their only interest is to "do good" for residents. But nonprofit organizations often give no more than their name and tax advantage to a nursing facility while its everyday management is handled by people who only work under contract with the organization. Even when the nonprofit organization takes an active role in running the facility—usually several facilities—there is no guarantee it will be any better at the job than profit-making managers. The test of care quality comes on the floor of the facility itself and not in the boardrooms of its owners.

Group Affiliation

Many nursing facilities are operated by or affiliated with religious, ethnic or fraternal organizations. Depending both on your interest and on the degree to which the affiliation affects daily life in the facility, this can be either good or bad. A particular affiliation may mean you and the other residents will have similar backgrounds and interests, which can make for a real feeling of community. Also, there may be specially targeted activities at the facility in which you will enjoy participating.

On the other hand, if a group or organization to which you do not belong dominates the social activity of a facility, it may make you an outsider and may also limit the availability of other, non-sectarian activities. Be aware of a facility's affiliation and its influence on daily life there.

2. Cost

Although it may generally be true that the more something costs, the better its quality, that is not necessarily the case with nursing facilities.

With nursing facilities, high price often means sophisticated and expensive medical equipment and staff. And although most residents will never need them, every resident winds up paying. Similarly, some facilities are expensive because they have to foot the bill for a shiny new building.

Many smaller, less expensive facilities with less high-tech equipment can provide a more comfortable setting with more individual attention and participation for residents. Of course, you must make certain that lower cost does not reflect a lack of essential services or of qualified personnel. But these are things to investigate and cannot be assumed from the cost of the care alone.

MORE IS NOT LESS

While one might guess that larger facilities cost less because they operate on an economy of scale, in general it is just the opposite. On the average, larger facilities cost more to operate than smaller ones, probably because of more and higher-level medical services and larger administrative staffs.

---

3. The Facility

Location

For a number of reasons, where a facility is located can be extremely significant. Continuing contact with people and life outside the facility is one of the residents' greatest concerns, and location can affect that contact in a number of ways.

Visiting. Can friends and relatives get there easily? Is it near public transportation? The ease with which people can visit has a direct bearing on how often they do.

Outings. Are there places nearby—a park, library, senior center—where elders can be taken for outings, either by visitors or by staff?

Immediate surroundings. Is the surrounding area noisy, peaceful, ugly, safe? What can be seen and heard through the windows during the day and night? Are short walks or a bit of lounging outside possible?

Number of Beds and Residents

As with most questions about nursing facilities, there is no simple guideline about whether a large or small one is best. It is mostly a matter of your own needs and tastes, and of the quality of care delivered. Of concern when assessing large facilities, those with over 100 beds, is whether their size means they're too institutional, too cold—and whether they still provide personal attention and permit residents to participate in their own care.

A small facility, on the other hand, may not have all the services and skilled personnel such as dieticians, rehabilitative therapists, and social workers, that a larger one has. But smaller facilities tend to be more personal and homey and allow residents greater control over their own daily lives.

The Facility's "Feel"

What is your first impression when you walk through the door? It may be the same general impression, conscious or unconscious, that a resident has all the time.

Homeyness. A facility should be as unlike a hospital as is consistent with good health care. It should be colorful, with personal, individual touches on walls and tables. Some facilities encourage residents to decorate their rooms and common areas; others have regulations against it. There should also be plenty of light, both from windows and lamps.

Healthfulness. The facility should be clean and free from strong odors. Infections and viruses pass easily in group living situations, and they can be very serious for elders. The space should not feel cramped; crowding is both physically and psychologically unhealthy. And the air should not be too hot, too cold, or too stuffy.

Odors may mean that food, linen, residents' clothing or personal hygiene are not being tended to often enough.

CHECK THE INSPECTION REPORT

Every nursing facility is inspected by state health care officials about once a year. The inspectors check for violations of state and federal health, safety and care standards. The state agency then describes those violations, along with residents' complaints, in a written report called a State Inspection Report or Compliance Survey. All facilities are supposed to make the report readily available to the public. Most good facilities will post the report on a bulletin board and have other copies available.

Read a facility's latest report carefully. Even the best among them will have some minor violations or complaints from residents. But a report that mentions many serious health violations, or repeated neglect of residents, should raise a red flag to you. The administrators at a facility should be willing to discuss the report with you and to explain what they are doing to address violations and complaints.

While a bad report means the facility has some explaining to do, a good report does not mean everything is hunky dory. Most facilities know roughly when an inspection is due—and some load up with extra staff to bring the facility up to par just for that time, then sink back to fewer staff and poorer conditions right after the inspection. When evaluating a facility, depend first and foremost on your own inspection.

Public Areas

Prospective residents often pay much less attention to common rooms than to residents' private rooms. But the comfort and attraction of the public areas affect the amount of time a resident spends out of his or her room, out of bed, and so may have a bearing on how active the resident remains. The following are some of the things you might consider.

A quiet room. Although one advantage of a nursing facility is that residents do not spend too much time alone, it can also be a problem. Most residents share rooms, and privacy can sometimes be difficult to find. It's important that some room or area is available for solitude or at least quiet—where there is no radio, television or group activities and where it is understood that people are to be left to themselves.

Eating areas. Food and rules about eating are discussed more fully below, but you should spend time both where food is served and eaten—dining room, private rooms, other areas of the facility—while residents are actually eating and, if possible, eat at least one, and if possible, two or three meals there with the residents.

Social, TV and activity rooms. While television can be good company for facility residents, it can also become a real annoyance. If there are televisions in all common areas, and they are always on, that can interfere with other activities, such as having a simple conversation. And if there are TVs on in all the common areas, that may signal that the staff is using the machines as distractions rather than interacting with the residents. Whether or not there is a "quiet" room, it should be possible to socialize somewhere without a TV blaring.

The social and activity rooms should be clean and comfortable and should have some personal touches. A simple way to tell whether the residents find these common rooms inviting is to see how many people are using them.

Outside areas. Is there a courtyard or other outside area where residents can spend time? Is there a garden in which residents can work? Both the air and change of scene from inside can be very refreshing to residents.

Visiting areas. Is there a place other than the resident's room for private visits? Must visiting take place in a room used for other purposes as well? Does the facility encourage visiting or make it seem like a bother?

Residents' Private Rooms

Many people who enter a nursing facility have not shared a room with anyone else for a long time, yet virtually all nursing facilities provide only double or triple rooms. Adjusting to the loss of privacy and need for compromise that go with sharing a bedroom can be difficult. The set-up and rules of the facility can make this transition either easier or harder. The following list suggests some things to look for:

Size. Are there single rooms, double, or triple? Are there adjoining bathrooms? Are the bathrooms set up to ensure privacy?

Light. Is there a window that lets in natural light? Are there individual reading lights near each bed? Can the lights be used without disturbing a roommate's sleep?

Structure. Does the set-up of the room, furniture and perhaps a curtain between beds allow some privacy for each roommate? Is there someplace to sit other than on the bed? Are there places for visitors to sit and visit privately? Can furnishings be moved around?

Security. Theft is a common problem in nursing facilities. Is there a place where personal possessions can be kept safely and easily retrieved? Is there a call button within reach of each bed that connects to the central aide station and can only be turned off at the bed?

Comfort. Is private furniture allowed in the room? Is room temperature controlled by each room? Are telephones, radios or televisions permitted in the rooms? If so, what are the rules to protect roommates from too much noise?

GETTING HELP FROM AN OMBUDSMAN

Every nursing facility has one or two people called ombudsmen who act as advocates for residents and their families when conflicts arise about facility rules or with facility staff. These ombudsmen are usually volunteers or employees of the state or county, not hired or paid by the facility. As independent observers, ombudsmen should be able to provide you with good, unbiased opinions about the quality of a particular nursing facility you are considering. And because an ombudsman usually works at more than one facility, he or she will probably be able to compare one facility with others in the area.

The operators of the nursing facility can give you the name and phone number of the local ombudsman for that facility, or let you know when he or she is slated to visit. The local ombudsman can then, in private, give you a picture of the facility and its staff, compare it with other area facilities and discuss whether the facility is particularly good or bad with residents who have similar physical or mental capabilities.

There is also a state ombudsman who oversees the local programs and who tracks formal complaints and health and safety violations against nursing facilities. If you call the state office, it may be willing to give you an overall assessment of several facilities you are considering. (See the Appendix for contact information.)

---

4. Services and Activities

Nursing facilities do not all offer the same services and activities beyond basic personal and medical care. Some facilities focus on exercise and therapy for physical impairments, others on social or educational programs, still others on developing residents' independence and memory. It is important to match services and activities with needs. For example, if a resident does not have the physical or mental capacity to be very active, recreational and social programs may be much less important than the amount of personal staff attention to cleanliness, comfort and conversation. For more active residents, though, activities that encourage independent thought and movement may be crucial to maintaining the highest possible levels of health.

Matching services and activities with needs cannot be done entirely in advance because it's difficult to anticipate what needs will be most important. Also, needs change over time. Try to choose a facility that encourages resident input into services and activities, and is attentive to a resident's individual needs. Discuss the flexibility of services and activities with the staff and listen for indications that residents' dignity, independence and individual differences are important.

Rehabilitation Therapy

Is the particular physical, respiratory, speech or other therapy you need regularly available in the facility or must special arrangements be made? Does the resident have to go outside the facility to receive the therapy? Is there extra cost?

WHAT YOU CAN LEARN FROM CONSULTING CARE PLANS

By law, a nursing facility must develop a written care plan for each resident. This plan includes an assessment of the resident's physical and cognitive abilities and needs, as well as his or her personality and social skills. Based on that assessment, the facility develops a plan for care, which should include: nursing, therapy and physical and memory exercise required; prescribed medications, plus medicine combinations to be avoided; social activities the resident favors and is able to join; and nutrition needs, including dietary restrictions and required eating assistance.

When considering a facility, ask to see some of the resident care plans that have recently been developed. Privacy need not be an issue; names can easily be blackened out in a copy. The plans should be tailored to meet each resident's individual limitations and needs; they should not all look the same. Also, ask about the facility's procedures for regularly updating the plans. And ask to see samples of plans that have been changed to meet a resident's changing condition and needs.

Social Activities and Other Services

The greatest concern of many nursing facility residents is for contact with the outside world—seeing family and other visitors, physically leaving the facility, receiving news, phone calls and mail.

Outings. Does the facility regularly organize outings to places and activities such as the library, park, local senior center, shopping? Is transportation provided? Are escorts available for a simple walk?

Incoming activity. Are visiting speakers and activities scheduled regularly? Is there a program of outside volunteers who participate with residents in some program or activity?

Organized events. Look at the facility's weekly or monthly calendar of events. Is there stimulation for mind and body—education, information and exercise—as well as just entertainment? Do organized activities take place in the evening as well as the day? Do people from outside the facility participate?

Personal care. Are there services for personal grooming and cleanliness, such as a visiting barber or hairdresser and a way to have clothes washed and cleaned? Does a dentist or dental hygienist visit the facility?

Social service assistance. Is there a counselor or social worker who can assist with family problems, paperwork, financial organization and referrals for outside services?

Facility-Wide Rules

Every facility has rules by which all residents and visitors must abide. Do they seem reasonable? Do the administrators seem willing to be flexible with those rules to meet individual needs? Ask to see the written rules and also try to find out about important rules of daily life which are not listed.

Visiting. When and where is visiting allowed? Are there any particular rules about children? What about phone calls in and out? Can visitors eat facility meals with residents?

Meals. Are mealtimes flexible? If a meal is missed, is there other food available to eat? Must meals be eaten in the dining area? Is food from outside the facility allowed?

Hours. Is there a set time when all residents are awakened? Is there a rule about having to get dressed? About going to bed? Watching television? Lights out? Is there a curfew for residents who have gone on an outing?

Bathing. If a resident needs assistance bathing, does he or she retain a reasonable choice about when and how often?

Privacy. Can a resident keep the private room door closed at will, or only during night hours? Must staff knock before entering? Is there privacy in the bathroom?

Privately hired aides. Some facilities allow residents to supplement the personal care staff with privately hired aides. This flexibility may be a good thing, but be wary if the practice is common. It may mean the staff relies on the outside aides and gives less care and personal attention to residents.

Medication Control

Over-medication is a serious problem for many older people—particularly for nursing facility residents. If several different medications are required, keeping track of them is sometimes difficult.

Some nursing facilities also encourage residents to take "as-needed" medication—sedatives, relaxants, sleeping medicines—instead of responding to their needs. It is important to note whether a facility monitors residents' medication carefully. The facility should:

- keep a written record for the personal physician and family to review;
- have a policy of periodic review of all medications a resident is taking;
- have a policy that any new medication shall be cleared in writing with a responsible family member; and
- have a clearly stated rule about the residents' right to refuse unwanted medication.

SPECIAL WARNING ON DRUG USE AND RESTRAINTS

A few nursing facilities prescribe and administer psychotropic drugs, also known as "chemical straightjackets." These drugs make residents easy for the facility to care for because, in essence, they turn active residents into zombies. Not only do these drugs rob residents of their humanity while they're directly under the influence, but they can do lasting physical and emotional damage as well.

Any good nursing facility should be willing to show you its written policy on psychotropic drugs. The policy should specify that no such drugs can be administered to a resident without the written consent of either the resident or certain designated family members, that any such written consent be for a limited period of time and that the designated family members and the resident's physician be notified of the administration of any such drugs.

There are legal limits on the use of restraints to hold a resident in a bed or chair. And both health care experts and nursing facility advocates seriously frown on the practice. Although in some limited circumstances restraints may be necessary for people who are in danger of falling if left unattended, some facilities use restraints like psychoactive drugs merely to "manage" residents who require more attention than the facility wants to give. Make sure to find out what the facility's policy is on the use of restraints. It should be clearly stated, should permit restraints only when the resident presents an immediate danger of physical injury to himself or herself or to others, and should require that a designated family member be notified when restraints are to be used.

Medical Records

Although technically required to keep records only of certain medical and nursing procedures they provide, a thorough nursing facility will also keep a written record of a resident's medical condition and of outside treatment by doctors, clinics and hospitals. It can be very helpful to a resident and to his or her physician if the facility keeps a written record of health problems that have not warranted medical treatment but have affected the resident's comfort and well-being— such as problems with elimination, digestion or sleeping, depression, too much time in bed, bedsores, eating problems or weight changes.

5. Other Residents

When considering a nursing facility, try to make several visits there and speak to some of the residents as you consider the matters discussed below.

Similar Levels of Care

Small facilities should admit only residents with relatively similar care needs; large facilities should provide only one level of care in each separate area or wing. There are several reasons for this. First, when care is kept to one level, personnel can be specialized; they may be better at what they do if they have fewer things to do. Costs may also be kept down because residents aren't paying for services they don't need.

There are also less tangible reasons for wanting to be with people whose needs are similar to your own. Residents can share their concerns and their ways of coping with common problems. Also, they need not be confronted daily with problems much different or more severe than their own. This is particularly important where mental orientation or capacity is concerned. Good facilities may separate the rooms of severe Alzheimer's or other dementia sufferers from the rooms of other residents. And when all the residents are together, the staff should pay special attention to residents who are disoriented.

Room Assignment

Most nursing facilities have two beds per room; some larger facilities have three. A few facilities offer private rooms, but they are very expensive. And a few small facilities have only private rooms. In surveys of residents, roommate selection ranks right behind contact with friends and relatives as most important.

Whatever your preference, find out whether the facility will take it into account in assigning a roommate. Some people prefer to have a roommate in similar physical condition so that they can better understand each other's needs and concerns. Other people do not mind having a roommate with greater needs; it allows them to be of help. Still others would prefer a roommate in better physical condition so that they can receive extra help.

There is also the matter of finding someone with common interests, religious or ethnic background, language and habits—smoking or late nights, for example. Will the facility consider these things when assigning a roommate? If so, make sure to let them know the things that are most important to you.

Residents' Condition and Activity

You can tell a lot about a nursing facility simply by walking around and looking carefully at the residents. Are most extremely ill or disabled? Do people appear comfortable? Are they reasonably neat and clean? Do you see smiles, hear friendly conversation among residents and between residents and staff? Are residents moving about the facility and being active in some way, or are they mostly in their rooms? Are people sitting alone and unattended in chairs or in hallways in wheelchairs?

By checking the common areas, you can tell whether the residents are doing things together or only on their own. It may take several visits, at different times of the day, to get a feel for this. Are there any ongoing communal activities, such as a newsletter, a garden, regular outings, some volunteer project? Be sure to ask.

6. Staff

As with judgments about residents, getting a sense of the staff requires spending some time at the facility during a normal day's activities.

Personal Care Aides

In virtually every nursing facility, 90% of direct resident care is provided by personal care aides—also called assistants, attendants or orderlies. These are the foot soldiers of nursing facility care, and their competence and attitude are most important to the health and well-being of residents. There are several things to find out about them.

Numbers. Although there are no hard and fast rules about how many attendants there should be for each resident, there must be enough so that the residents receive attention most of the time when they want it, and any time they need it. Generally, a good facility will have one aide on duty in a given wing or section of a facility for every five or six residents there. At night, the figure may drop to one aide for every 15 or so residents. On the other hand, during meals, when resident needs are high, aides should be supplemented by nurses, volunteers or other assistants so that there is one person to help every three or four people. In addition to these numbers, use your eyes to judge whether there is enough staff: Are there residents who seem to want attention from an aide but are not getting it?

Turnover. How long have people worked at the facility? Long-term employment generally means that both aides and residents are satisfied with the aides' work. A rapid turnover of aides may be a bad sign, although even the best facilities sometimes have a hard time keeping staff, particularly in the aide jobs, which are usually high in stress and low in pay.

Language. If English is not the first language of the resident, how many people on the staff speak the resident's first language? The reverse may also be true: What percentage of the staff speaks understandable English?

Intangibles. The importance of the courtesy, friendliness and efficiency of the personal care aides to both residents and visitors cannot be overemphasized. But the only way to judge this is to see the aides and residents in their daily interchanges. Is there easy conversation? Do the aides seem to pay attention to what the residents want? Do the aides have a neat and professional appearance?

Remember, as with any group of people, not every aide and every resident are going to get along. The crucial thing is not that every interaction is smiling and efficient, but that most contacts are cordial and responsive to a resident's needs.

Available Professional Staff

The number of personnel listed on stationery with impressive certificates and licenses matters very little. What counts is how much time any of them actually spends with residents. How often does the facility's physician check on medical care standards? How often do licensed nurses make rounds? How easy is it to schedule a rehabilitation therapist? How much hands-on care do the professional level personnel provide and how much are they just supervising? To what extent can a resident request direct care from one of the professional staff?

Direct physician care will, except in emergencies, come from your own physicians, not from the facility's doctors. Find out whether the facility restricts visits from outside physicians and whether it provides transportation to outside medical appointments. Also, many physicians will not make visits to a nursing facility. Ask whether your primary care physician will make such visits, and if so, whether he or she includes the particular facility you have in mind.

Outside Help

Find out whether the facility permits or arranges for extra outside help.

Volunteers. Many facilities make good use of volunteers from public service agencies and programs. Some simply provide extra personal attention or companionship, while others bring special educational skills or social programs. These volunteers are a good link to the outside world and give residents a change of pace and face from the regular staff.

Private aid. Does the facility allow part-time private assistance of any sort from outside the facility, such as a private duty care assistant, chiropractor, massage therapist or private duty nurse?

7. Food

In a nursing facility, the importance of meals goes beyond merely getting the right nutrients. Meals are central activities in a resident's day—a social event and a source of pleasure when many other events and pleasures are no longer available. In inquiring about a facility's food service, don't restrict yourself to looking at a menu or seeing that a dietician is an official member of the staff. Instead, visit the facility's dining areas during one or more meals, and eat the food with residents. There are several things to ask, look and taste for.

Tastiness. Simple truths are often overlooked, such as the fact that the nutritional value of food is wasted if the food is not eaten. Another is that if food tastes lousy, people eat less of it. Freshness and variety also help keep people interested. Check menus from a week or two and see how often fresh foods are served and how often dishes are repeated.

Preferences and restrictions. No group living facility can cater to the different food whims and desires of all its residents. But residents should be offered some choice in meals, and the facility should respond to strong likes and dislikes. Dietary restrictions, whether for health, digestive or religious reasons, must be strictly followed. The facility should keep a written record of any such restriction for each resident, and the kitchen staff should consult it before, not after, planning and preparing meals.

Extra food. Not everyone's appetite runs by the standard meal clock. Some people prefer, or need, to eat a little bit several times a day. Other people who are up at "odd" hours get hungry. And many people get pleasure from special foods made by friends or relatives or a favorite neighborhood bakery. A facility that is too rigid about food is not taking care of important needs.

Does the facility serve snacks, tea or coffee between meals, or at least make such things available to residents? Do the snacks include fresh fruit and other healthful foods? May residents eat the snacks where and when they want—particularly, in their own rooms—or only at designated times and places? May residents be given food from outside the facility? And if so, is there an easily accessible place in which to keep it fresh?

Dining area. The first thing to pay attention to when you visit the dining area during a meal is whether the residents are eating the food. That will tell you a lot. Observe whether the staff is helpful with residents who need assistance eating. Are residents comfortable and is the area clean? Ask if dining times are flexible. Do residents have enough time with their meal or is food rushed in and out?

8. Family Involvement

Although one benefit of a nursing facility is its ready-made community of companions and helpers, there are important benefits in active family involvement in the resident's life. Residents rate personal contact—by visits, phone, mail and outings—at the top of their list of concerns. And no matter how good a facility's own outreach programs are, a resident's ability to stay in touch with the larger community requires help from friends and relatives.

Whether family and friends are actively involved in a resident's life depends to no small degree on whether the facility encourages their participation. Families should be regularly invited to participate in activities with residents. Visiting should be encouraged rather than merely tolerated. Therefore, there should be adequate space, comfort and privacy in visiting areas and wide and flexible visiting hours. Visiting should be permitted during meals and there should be wide latitude in taking residents for outings.

Together, the staff and resident's family should regularly review the resident's condition and care. Find out what the procedures are for family consultation about problems or changes in the resident's care plan or room or roommate assignment. Another thing to ask about is whether there is an organized family support group or network which keeps residents' families in touch with one another.

9. Decision-Making

Residents' long-term health and comfort directly depend on a facility's procedures for making decisions about their care. A good facility should have standardized procedures about residents' daily care decisions. Review them before deciding about a particular facility. If a facility refuses to respond to a resident's complaints, there are state and local government agencies which can step in. See the discussion of the Nursing Facility Ombudsman, below.

Residents' Problems and Complaints

It is a sad but widely recognized truth that there is significant patient abuse and neglect in nursing facilities. And there are also many smaller problems that, if unattended, can make a resident's life miserable. It is therefore very important that there are specific procedures for residents and family members to lodge a complaint or discuss a problem about a particular staff person, a method or type of care, or a facility rule or condition.

The danger of not having an explicit complaint procedure is that a resident will not know with whom to speak, or will get a runaround from staff members who claim they have no authority to do anything to right the wrong. Find out how complaints are handled and make certain that the process guarantees a response from an identifiable person in authority.

Similarly, there should be a regular procedure to register a complaint or discuss a problem about a roommate or other resident. Find out what these procedures are, and what needs to be done to make a room change at the resident's request.

Facility-Imposed Changes

For financial and other reasons, when there are vacancies in double rooms, a facility may want to move residents around. Or, because of a change in a resident's condition that requires a different level of care, the facility may believe a room change is necessary. However, the resident may disagree. It is therefore important that a resident have a right to be notified in advance of a change, and that the facility have rules that limit the circumstances under which such changes can be made.

As with a room change, the facility may decide that the particular non-medical care a resident has been receiving is no longer necessary, or that new types of costlier or more restrictive care are required.

Find out how these decisions are made and what rights the resident has regarding them. Also make sure there is a provision for consultation and notification of the family.

For all decisions about medical care or changes in condition, specific written procedures should be set out, including:

- what decisions can be made by aides and what must be decided by the nurse on duty;
- when the facility's attending physician must be consulted about a change in medical care or condition;
- when the resident's personal physician must be consulted about a change in condition or a possible change in care;
- when the resident's family must be notified of a change in care or condition.

Nursing Facility Ombudsman

The federal government funds a program, administered by each state's Agency on Aging, which makes available to nursing facility residents an ombudsman—a kind of trouble-shooter to mediate unresolved problems between residents or their families and a nursing facility. The ombudsman has regular visiting hours and days at the facility and should also be available by phone. There is no charge to the resident for the services of the ombudsman.

C. Entering a Formal Residence Contract

All facilities have a formal written document which both you and a facility representative sign. It does not matter whether this document is called a "contract" or an "agreement" or something similar. What does matter is that all important terms and conditions of residence and care are included, so that both you and the facility are clear about them. If you are unsure of any terms and conditions, consider having an attorney or someone else familiar with nursing facility care review it with you before signing. Even if you do not consult with anyone else, take the agreement home and review it carefully before signing.

If something important to you is not included in the facility's pre-printed agreement, discuss it with the proper facility official, and when you've reached an agreement, write it on a separate piece of paper, signed and dated by both you and the facility official and attach it to the rest of the agreement.

1. What to Look for in a Written Agreement

The agreement should spell out the specific health care, personal care, equipment and supplies included in the level of care for which you are paying a regular daily, weekly or monthly fee. This should include frequency of nursing care and physical or other therapies, plus number of meals and special dietary needs.

Room. The agreement should specify the number of beds in the resident's room, as well as any other features that distinguish the type of room from others in the facility and are important to you—such as the room size, bathroom facilities, windows, location in the building.

Extra charges and adjustments. The agreement should specify what services, equipment and supplies are charged as extra—above the regular rate. The agreement should also specify amounts to be subtracted for such things as meals eaten outside of the facility and time spent away, such as vacations or time in the hospital.

Some contracts require that residents purchase their medications at the facility's own pharmacy. Since the rates there may be considerably higher than at outside pharmacies, this is in effect a forced extra charge. Find out in advance whether this is the policy at any facility you are considering.

Rate changes. The agreement should spell out whether, and how much, the regular rate will go up or down if the level of care is changed, whether the regular rate is guaranteed to remain the same for any length of time and how much notice must be given before rates are raised.

Change in funding. As discussed in Chapter 5, Medicare and private insurance coverage for nursing facility care is very limited. And Medicaid coverage, while extensive, is not available to everyone at all times. (See Chapter 6.) Also, some facilities provide certain rooms for Medicaid residents and other, better rooms for private paying patients, so that even if Medicaid begins to cover you at some point, you may be forced to move to a different, less desirable room to receive it.

It is very important to find out not only what your coverage is when entering the facility, but also what your personal financial responsibility would be, and how the facility would respond in changing circumstances such as:

- after your allotted Medicare skilled nursing facility coverage is used up;
- moving from skilled to intermediate or personal care, neither of which is covered by Medicare or private insurance;
- becoming eligible for Medicaid if the facility does not accept it;
- personal bankruptcy. Many facilities require proof of your ability to pay for two years as a condition of admission.

Discharge policy. There are situations in which either you anticipate moving out of the facility or the facility wants to discharge you even though you do not necessarily want to leave. Find out the facility's policies and procedures, including how much written notice must be given, in the following and any other discharge situations:

- if the resident's need for care changes and the resident wants to leave the facility to receive different care;

- if the resident's need for care changes and the facility wants the resident to move out and receive care elsewhere; and
- if the resident's source of funds changes.

CHECK THE POLICY ON TEMPORARY HOSPITALIZATION

It is not uncommon for a nursing facility resident to require hospitalization for some period of time. Find out what the policy is on holding a resident's bed during hospitalization. If you may be going back and forth to the hospital and you can too easily lose your place in the facility while hospitalized, you may not want that nursing facility. ■

Medicare and Veterans' Benefits

B race yourself for some serious numbers.
The cost of nursing facility care averages $3,500 to $5,000 per month—and some cost as much as $10,000 per month. Even the least expensive custodial-only care facilities average almost $3,000 per month. And these amounts are increasing much faster than the general cost of living. With such costs, most people exhaust their personal savings within six months of entering a residential care facility. Yet many long-term care residents stay in nursing facilities for two years or more, with total costs often reaching $100,000 to $200,000. Home health care, too, can run into thousands of dollars a year if services are skilled or frequent.

Who pays for all this? For the most part, the answer is: you pay. At least until all your money is gone, after which Medicaid may begin to pay. (See Chapter 6.) A widely held misconception about the Medicare system is that it "covers" nursing facility care. The truth is that Medicare pays only about two percent of all nursing facility costs. Medicare coverage for nursing facilities averages less than 30 days of care—and that applies only to skilled nursing care. Medicare covers no long-term nursing facility or other residential care, and its home health care coverage is equally limited.

Private long-term care insurance may pay some of the cost of nursing facility care. But even if you have such insurance, you may wind up having to pay so much that you will deplete your savings. (See Chapter 10.)

The only comprehensive coverage of long-term care comes from Medicaid. This federal government program for low-income people, administered by the states, pays for almost half the nation's total nursing facility costs and for much home care as well. But, as is discussed later (in Chapter 6), a person is not eligible for Medicaid coverage until he or she has used up almost all personal assets. In other words, if you have money saved when you begin long-term care, you must pay the bills yourself until your money is nearly gone; only then will Medicaid begin to pay.

If the alternative of home care is workable for you and your family, little of the cost will be covered by government programs or private insurance. Even so, your out-of-pocket expenses may be lower than for residential care. If you do enter a residential facility, the odds are that you will wind up personally paying for the bulk of care until your assets are nearly gone.

There is no easy way out of this staggering financial crunch. The task is to make your money last as long as possible. You want to be able to use your assets for things other than long-term care. And you want to maintain private assets as long as possible so that you can pay for long-term care services not covered by any government program or insurance.

Once you are actually faced with the need for long-term care, the best way to protect your assets is to get only the services or level of care you really need from the most cost-efficient provider. (See Chapters 1 through 4.) But be aware of how much and under what rules Medicare, the Veterans' Administration and Medicaid may pay for long-term care, so that you can get the most from these programs. And even long in advance of your need for long-term care, you may be able to take some steps to protect some of your assets. Long-term care insurance is one avenue. (See Chapter 10.) And transferring some of your assets to others may also save some money from long-term care costs.

A. Medicare Coverage for Long-Term Care

Most Americans 65 and older are eligible for Medicare coverage, but few understand how it works. Medicare is a federal government program formed to assist older Americans with medical costs. The program is divided into two parts: Part A is "hospital insurance," which covers some bills for a stay in a hospital or a skilled nursing facility; Part B is "medical insurance," which pays some of the costs of doctors and outpatient medical care. If you are 65 or older and eligible for Social Security retirement, survivor's or dependent's benefits, you are automatically eligible for Part A coverage. And for a monthly premium anyone 65 or older can enroll in Part B coverage, whether or not they are eligible for Part A.

FOR ADDITIONAL INFORMATION

Even people who are not eligible for Social Security benefits may be eligible for Part A Medicare when they reach age 65. For a complete discussion of how a person can become eligible for Medicare, see *Social Security, Medicare and Pensions: Get the Most Out of Your Retirement and Medical Benefits*, by Joseph Matthews with Dorothy Matthews Berman (Nolo).

One of the worst misconceptions about Medicare is that it covers nursing facility care. In fact, Medicare nursing facility coverage is severely limited and leaves most people to pay for virtually all long-term care out of their own pockets.

Because home health care can sometimes be considerably cheaper than nursing facility care, it would seem sensible for the government to encourage home care by covering a sizable portion of the cost. Unfortunately, it does not. Medicare pays much less of home care than such logic might lead you to expect, and pays nothing at all for residential care alternatives to nursing homes, such as personal care facilities.

Just as important as knowing what long-term care Medicare does pay for so you can get the most out of available coverage, is knowing what Medicare does not pay for so you can be prepared either to gather the funds from somewhere else or to obtain most of your care and coverage from other sources.

1. Skilled Nursing Facility Care

Part A of Medicare covers a small amount of skilled nursing facility care, as follows:

- up to 100 days per benefit period—which refers to a continuous period of treatment—in a skilled nursing facility;
- a semi-private room (two to four beds); if you want a private room, you must pay for the difference yourself, unless the private room is medically necessary as prescribed by a doctor and approved by the facility and the Medicare intermediary—an insurance company that administers Medicare funds in your state;
- daily, regular, skilled and special nursing as medically necessary, but *not* a private duty nurse;
- skilled rehabilitation services—such as physical, occupational or speech therapy—as medically necessary and as long as you are showing improvement; and
- medications, medical supplies and equipment, and dietary requirements as supplied by the facility.

WARNING—MEDICARE DOES NOT COVER

- custodial care (non-medical assistance with the normal daily activities such as eating and bathing) unless it is part of skilled nursing care in a skilled nursing facility;
- nursing care or therapy provided in a facility that is not certified by Medicare as a *skilled* nursing facility; or
- doctor's care while you are in a nursing facility. However, Medicare Part B "medical insurance" covers doctor's care in a nursing facility under the same terms as in any other situation.

Conditions Limiting Medicare Coverage

Unfortunately, the many conditions placed on Medicare coverage of nursing facility costs eliminate far more care than they cover. When you add these conditions to the fact that Medicare partially pays for a total of only 100 days, it is easy to understand why Medicare pays for only about two percent of all nursing facility costs.

Immediate prior hospital stay. Medicare pays for a stay in a skilled nursing facility only if you have first spent at least three consecutive days (not counting the discharge day) in a hospital. And you must be admitted to the nursing facility within 30 days of your discharge from the hospital.

Daily skilled nursing care or therapy. Medicare pays only for the skilled nursing care or rehabilitative therapy you need and receive every day. If you receive such care intermittently, you do not qualify for Medicare coverage because you fail to meet this requirement.

Prescribed by a physician. Your daily skilled nursing care or therapy must be "medically necessary"—specifically prescribed by a doctor.

Medicare-approved skilled nursing facility. You must receive care in a *skilled* nursing facility which is certified by Medicare. Medicare checks on the quality of care of each nursing facility and certifies those which meet its standards. Ask to see the current Medicare certification documents of any nursing facility you are considering. And care that is, or could be, received in a lower level facility is not covered.

Only while condition "improving." Even though Medicare could cover up to 100 days in a skilled nursing facility, and even though you may need daily skilled care for all those days, Medicare will cover you only as long as your condition is "improving." Once your condition has stabilized, according to review by Medicare (see below), it will no longer pay for skilled nursing facility care—no matter how serious your condition remains or how much skilled nursing care you continue to need.

Approval on review. The fact that your doctor prescribes "medically necessary" skilled nursing care for you in a skilled nursing facility, and continues to certify that your condition is improving, still does not guarantee that Medicare will provide nursing facility coverage. The doctor's opinion must be approved by both the nursing facility's Utilization Review Committee—facility doctors who review patient conditions—and by the Medicare "intermediary."

How Much Medicare Pays of Nursing Facility Costs

During the first 100 days of coverage, Medicare pays the amounts noted below.

Days 1 to 20. You are responsible for paying up to your yearly Medicare Part A deductible—if you have not already reached it. Once you have paid the yearly deductible, Medicare pays all your covered nursing facility charges.

Days 21 to 100. After the first 20 days of coverage, Medicare pays all covered charges except what is called a "coinsurance" amount, for which you are personally responsible. For 1999, that coinsurance amount was $96 per day; the figure goes up each year.

Days 101 on. After 100 days in a skilled nursing facility you are on your own. Medicare pays nothing toward your stay there.

2. Medicare Home Care Coverage

Although Medicare coverage for home care is extremely limited, it can provide substantial payment for the most expensive part of home care—skilled nursing or therapy—during the time immediately following an illness or injury, when you are most likely to need it.

Home Health Services Covered by Medicare

Medicare-covered home health care services are listed below, limited by the conditions discussed in the following section:

- skilled nursing;
- physical and speech therapy: as needed during recovery, while improving;
- supplemental care: if, and only if, you receive skilled nursing or physical or speech therapy, Medicare may also pay for limited visits by a home health care aide to help you with personal care— usually only if there is no one else at home to help. Medicare may also cover required medical social services, some medical supplies or equipment provided by the home care agency, and the services of an occupational therapist to help you relearn daily household tasks.

REMINDER

Medicare home health care does not cover custodial personal care, drugs, meals or homemaking services.

Restrictions on Home Health Care Coverage

As with nursing facility care, a number of restrictions limit home health care coverage. Medicare applies only during periods of recovery from acute illness or injury, or following a change in condition while you are learning how to administer drugs or otherwise care for yourself.

Intermittent skilled care. It must be "medically necessary" for you to receive skilled nursing care or rehabilitative therapy on a part-time only basis. Full-time nursing care at home is not covered. Note that this is the opposite of the requirement for such care in a skilled nursing facility.

Doctor-prescribed. The skilled care must have been ordered by a physician.

Only during recovery. Care is covered only while you are recovering—that is, while your condition is improving. As soon as your condition has stabilized, as determined by a Medicare review, coverage ends.

Injury, illness or medical condition. Your need for care must be the result of a specific injury, illness or medical condition. If it is the result of general frailness, Medicare will not cover home care.

Confined to home. Care is covered only while you are confined to home except for brief, infrequent occasions out, usually related to receiving medical care. "Confined to home" is defined as being unable to leave home without difficulty and without the assistance of another person or a medical device such as a wheelchair. Confined to home does not necessarily mean bedridden, however.

Approved agency. Care must be provided by a Medicare-certified home care agency or other provider. This sometimes eliminates independent nurses and therapists. Always ask the home care agency or other provider to show you its Medicare certification documentation before beginning care.

How Much Medicare Home Health Coverage Pays

In general, Medicare pays 100% of the "approved costs" of the covered services provided by a certified home care agency or other provider. "Approved costs" are the standardized charges Medicare decides are appropriate for specific services, based on a national cost average. You are personally responsible for the cost of any non-covered services such as homemaking or unapproved personal care from a home care aide.

No matter what the home care provider might normally charge for the covered services, it must accept as payment in full whatever Medicare decides is the approved cost. The home care agency will submit all bills for covered services directly to Medicare. You don't have to be involved in the paperwork.

In some situations, it may not be clear whether Medicare will cover a particular service. In that case, the home care agency or other provider must notify you in writing of that doubt before it provides the service. If it does notify you and you accept the service anyway but Medicare denies coverage, you are personally responsible for the bill. If it does not notify you in advance, the provider cannot bill you.

LONG-TERM CARE COVERAGE BY HMOS AND MEDI-GAP INSURANCE

Many people have private health insurance that supplements their Medicare coverage, commonly called medi-gap. Many others get Medicare coverage through membership in an HMO or other managed care plan. Most medi-gap and managed care plans cover no more of nursing facility or home health care than Medicare. If Medicare does not cover it, a medi-gap policy or managed care plan usually does not cover it, either. And medi-gap or managed care payments plus Medicare's payments may still leave some part of the bills unpaid—even for covered care.

A few managed care plans do offer extra home care and nursing care coverage beyond what Medicare covers. This coverage is not for long-term care, but it may pay for a few extra weeks. And given the cost of nursing facility and home care, even a few weeks of coverage is worth collecting.

B. Veterans' Benefits for Long-Term Care

The Veterans' Administration operates more than 150 hospitals and a number of outpatient clinics throughout the United States that provide free or very low-cost health care for veterans and their dependents. The care at these facilities is usually very good, but in-patient care is limited. Although there are many hospitals and over 100,000 beds, there are millions of veterans and their dependents, so the VA reserves in-patient care for the treatment of acute conditions, with priority to service-connected illness and injury and to veterans who cannot afford care elsewhere. Some space for in-patient long-term care for the elderly is available, but it is severely limited.

1. Eligibility for Veterans' Benefits

Many elders may be eligible for Veterans' Administration medical benefits based on their military service or their spouse's service even if their current need for long-term care has nothing to do with any service connected disability. Disability compensation for "service-connected disability" and pension benefits for financially needy veterans are not discussed here, but may be available as extra sources of income. Check with your local Veterans' Administration for eligibility.

In general, any veteran is eligible for medical care from a VA facility if unable to afford care elsewhere. Dependents and survivors of veterans with service-connected disabilities, or those who receive veterans' pensions or are eligible for Medicaid, are also eligible to receive medical care from VA facilities if they are unable to afford the care elsewhere.

2. Home Health Care Covered by Veterans' Benefits

There are more and more home health care units connected to Veterans' Administration hospitals and clinics. And the care is free of charge. But unless there is such a home care unit in your area, the VA will rarely pay for care provided by an outside agency.

If a VA facility near you has a home health care unit, it can provide complete medical and personal care as often as necessary. The period of care is usually limited to recovery from acute illness, injury or surgery, but if specific medical care is needed, it may be available on a long-term basis.

So, if you are a veteran or dependent or survivor of a veteran who needs home health care, contact your local VA office to find out if home care is available from a facility in your area. If it is, it may well be worth finding out about eligibility and coverage.

3. Nursing Facility Care Covered by Veterans' Benefits

A number of VA facilities provide long-term skilled nursing and intermediate residential care for veterans. In general, simple custodial care without the need for regular nursing or other health care is not available, but where the VA draws the line in a given case may depend on the availability of beds in a particular facility.

VA coverage for skilled or intermediate care in a private facility is sometimes possible if similar care is not available in a VA facility. Eligibility depends on financial need as well as any connection between the disability or impairment and military service. Because the quality of free VA health care tends to be very good while costing the veteran nothing, it is worth it to investigate both your eligibility and the availability of long-term residential care in a VA facility. The search for information should begin with your local VA office and with any VA medical facility in your area. ■

Medicaid Coverage for Long-Term Care

Medicaid, or Medi-Cal in California, is a federally funded program, administered by the individual states, which helps pay for medical care for financially needy people. For low-income older people who qualify, Medicaid supplements Medicare to cover many long-term costs Medicare does not—including home care and almost all levels of nursing facility care for an unlimited time. The Medicaid program pays for about half of the country's total nursing facility costs.

To qualify for Medicaid, an elder must have a low income and very few assets. Unfortunately, this means that many people are not eligible until they have used up almost all their savings paying for nursing facility or home care themselves.

Another problem with Medicaid nursing facility coverage is that many facilities either do not accept Medicaid residents, or put them only in less desirable rooms, because Medicaid pays a lower rate than that charged to privately paying residents. So, if you are dependent on Medicaid when you enter a nursing facility, your choices may be limited. And if your funds diminish to the point that you become eligible for Medicaid after you are a resident, although by law the facility cannot discharge you, it might move you to a different room. Before choosing a nursing facility, find out the details of its Medicaid policy.

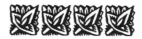

A NOTE ON FINANCIAL PLANNING

As discussed below, Medicaid is a program intended to help people who have low income and few assets. Its rules severely restrict the amount of savings one can keep and still be eligible for coverage. Rules also prevent people from merely moving their money around to skirt the rules for Medicaid eligibility.

There are, however, a few options available to people who are likely to need Medicaid coverage for long-term care and who have slightly too many assets to qualify for Medicaid—or who want to try to keep at least some of their assets to pass on to their survivors. These options may require advance planning. And some require that the older person must give up control over some assets. So, for many people, these alternatives are not practical or attractive. Even with these limitations, however, you should at least learn about these possible options, and do so as early as possible. (See Chapter 7.)

A. Eligibility for Medicaid

Each state has its own Medicaid eligibility standards, so check with your county's social services agency for the rules in your state. Overall federal government standards require your assets and income to be below certain levels, with special rules for nursing facility residents, which differ greatly for married couples and unmarried individuals. Note that for Medicaid purposes, the term unmarried includes divorced people and those whose spouse is no longer living.

1. Home Care: Income and Asset Limits

The following are the general federal guidelines for the amount of income and assets—savings, investment, property—a person receiving care who is not a resident of a nursing facility is allowed to keep and still receive Medicaid funds. Some states have stricter rules, other states are more liberal. If you are close to these figures, be sure to apply.

Income limits

An individual can have a monthly income of around $300 to $500 and still qualify for Medicaid; for a couple, the figure is roughly $500 to $700. Income includes Social Security and other government benefits, wages or self-employment income, interest or dividends from savings and investments, rents, royalties, pensions, annuities and gifts. If one spouse is still working, though, the first $65 per month of earned income (wages or self-employment) plus one-half of all amounts over that is not counted toward these income limits.

Asset limits

People who are not residents of a nursing facility may have non-exempt assets of no more than $2,000 ($3,000 for a couple). Fortunately, a number of assets are exempted from these figures. The most significant exempt asset is your home, if either you or your spouse live in it. Also exempted are your car up to a value of $4,500 and up to $2,000 worth of household goods and personal effects. Again, these are approximate figures and you must check with your local county social services office to find out the specific rules in your state.

Whose Money Counts?

Medicaid has a number of rules for counting assets and income to determine eligibility:

- The assets and income of children, grandchildren or other relatives do not count toward Medicaid limits, even if they live in the same household as the elder applying for Medicaid, except to the extent they provide regular financial support. Regular financial support is not limited to money but can include food and clothing or other personal items.
- If a married couple live together, both of their incomes and assets are counted toward the Medicaid limits.
- If a couple is divorced or legally separated and living apart, then only the income and assets of the spouse applying for Medicaid are counted, including any actual support received from the other spouse.
- If a couple live together but are not married, only the income and assets of the person applying for Medicaid are counted, including any direct financial support received from the other partner.

MEDICAID MAY PAY FOR ASSISTED LIVING

A few states are beginning to experiment with Medicaid coverage for some assisted living as well as for nursing facilities. Where coverage is available, it is only for people in assisted living who require nursing care. The rules pertaining to Medicaid eligibility for assisted living residents are the same as for people in nursing facilities.

For a complete discussion of assisted living as an alternative to nursing facility care, see Chapter 3, Section B. To find out whether Medicaid covers assisted living in some parts of your state, see Section C of this chapter.

---

2. Special Nursing Facility Medicaid Rules

Once a nursing facility resident has qualified, Medicaid pays virtually all facility costs for as long as a person remains there. But as with home care, a nursing facility resident is only eligible when his or her assets are below a certain level. Until then, the resident must pay. Once Medicaid begins paying, almost all of an individual's or a couple's income will go to the nursing home to reduce the amounts Medicaid pays.

Because Medicaid rules for nursing facility residents are quite different for unmarried individuals and for couples, this section is divided in two parts. The first section explains the income and assets which can be retained by a single person who enters a nursing facility. The second section explains the income and assets that each member of a married couple can retain when one spouse enters a nursing facility.

Unmarried Individuals in a Nursing Facility

Remember that for Medicaid purposes, "unmarried" includes those who are divorced or whose spouse has died. Also, beware that if your marital status changes after you qualify for Medicaid, the Medicaid limits on your income and assets will also change.

Income Eligibility Limits

About 30 states have no limits at all on the income a nursing facility resident can have and still be eligible for Medicaid coverage. But note that, as discussed below, virtually all of that income will go to the nursing facility, with Medicaid paying the balance of the cost.

The rest of the states do have eligibility income limits, which vary from about $700 to $1,100 per month. A nursing facility resident in one of these states with an income over the limit does not qualify for Medicaid coverage at all.

STATES WITH INCOME TEST FOR MEDICAID ELIGIBILITY

Alabama	Florida	Nevada	South Dakota
Alaska	Georgia	New Jersey	Tennessee
Arkansas	Idaho	New Mexico	Texas
Colorado	Iowa	Oklahoma	Wyoming
Delaware	Louisiana	South Carolina	

Income Retained by the Resident

If an unmarried nursing facility resident qualifies for Medicaid, all of that person's monthly income will go to the nursing facility, with Medicaid paying the balance of the nursing facility bill, except:

- A small monthly amount for personal needs—books and magazines, grooming and toilet articles—with the total value ranging from $30 to $70, depending on the state.
- Credit is given toward the nursing facility bill for income the resident spends directly on Medicare premiums, deductibles and co-payments, on medical insurance and on out-of-pocket medical expenses not covered by Medicare or Medicaid.
- In about 30 states, a resident can keep $150 to $600 a month for upkeep and repairs on his or her private residence. This home maintenance allowance is permitted for up to six months upon a written prognosis by the resident's doctor that the resident is expected to be able to return home from the nursing facility within six months after entering it.

Asset Eligibility Limits

Before Medicaid will cover an unmarried person's stay in a nursing facility, that person's savings and other assets must be reduced to certain limits. If your assets exceed these limits, you will qualify for Medicaid coverage only after you have paid for nursing facility coverage out of your own pocket—referred to by Medicaid as "spending down"—until you reach these limits. The Medicaid limits allow:

- no more than $2,000 in savings or other liquid assets such as stocks or certificates of deposit. This limit varies slightly from state to state;

- household and personal items up to a value of about $2,000;

- one automobile up to a value of $4,500;

- one wedding and one engagement ring of any value;

- a burial plot and up to $1,500 in a separately maintained fund for burial costs;

- a life insurance policy with a face value of no more than $1,500;

- a home, under limited circumstances. In some states, a home will not be counted in determining Medicaid eligibility for nursing facility coverage only if your doctor certifies in writing that you are likely to recover sufficiently to leave the nursing facility and return home. Some states also add a six-month to twelve-month time limit, no matter what your doctor says. In other states, your home remains exempt if you merely indicate on your nursing facility admission form that you intend to return home; even if the chances of returning are remote, you must indicate your intent to do so to qualify for this exemption.

Note that Medicaid rules do not permit you to simply give away assets to relatives or friends and then qualify for coverage. The few permissible methods to protect some assets are discussed in detail in Chapter 7.

HOW DOES MEDICAID KNOW WHAT YOUR ASSETS ARE?

A natural question arises when people read that Medicaid coverage is available only to people whose assets are below certain levels: How does Medicaid know what my assets are?

The answer is that when you apply for Medicaid, you fill out extensive application forms that ask you to list all your assets. You must also show the Medicaid eligibility workers copies of all ownership documents, bank books and the like. If there are any large or regular withdrawals from your assets in the 36 months prior to your application, you will have to prove where that money went and why. Remember, too, that Medicaid will have your Social Security number, so it can cross-check many financial transactions. Medicaid eligibility workers can also pay home visits.

If you fail to report income or assets and are caught by Medicaid, you run the risk of being denied coverage, being forced to repay any money already paid on your behalf and even facing criminal and civil penalties.

Married Couples with One Spouse in a Nursing Facility

While most states do not set income limits for unmarried people entering a nursing facility, there are different rules for couples. Many states set limits for couples when one spouse is in a nursing facility.

Whose Income Counts for Eligibility?

Most states use a "name-on-the-check" rule to determine whether income received by a married couple is counted against the Medicaid eligibility of the spouse in the nursing facility. This rule basically says that if the income is received solely in the name of the at-home spouse, it is not counted toward the state's maximum income limit for the nursing facility spouse's Medicaid eligibility.

Two states—California and Washington—have "community property" rules which can help a nursing facility spouse qualify for Medicaid coverage when the name-on-the-check rule would deny eligibility. If the nursing facility spouse in a community property state receives income in his or her name that is over the state's Medicaid limit, Medicaid will see how much income is received in the name of the at-home spouse as well. If one-half the total community property income (the combined income received in the name of both spouses) is not over the limit, then the nursing facility spouse will qualify for Medicaid even though the name-on-the-check rule would have denied eligibility.

Three other states—Indiana, Nebraska and West Virginia—also count the at-home spouse's income over certain limits as part of the nursing facility spouse's income when calculating eligibility.

Income Retained by Each Spouse

Of income received in his or her own name, the nursing facility spouse may keep between $30 to $70 per month for personal use, plus amounts to pay for Medicare, other medical insurance and medical expenses not covered by Medicare or Medicaid. The rest of the income in the name of the nursing facility spouse goes to the nursing facility, except for an amount needed to meet the at-home spouse's minimum allowance. The at-home spouse is allowed to keep all income in his or her own name. If more than half the couple's joint income is in the nursing facility spouse's name, the at-home spouse is allowed to keep some of the income in the nursing facility spouse's name up to a basic living allowance of between $1,000 and $2,000 per month, combining the two incomes. The specific amount varies from state to state. Check with the local social services agency to find out the limits in your state.

Assets Retained by Both Spouses

The name-on-the-check rule does not apply to assets—savings, property, investments. It used to be true that if a couple transferred all their assets to the sole name of the at-home spouse, the nursing facility spouse might qualify for Medicaid. No longer. Medicaid now looks at the combined assets of both spouses, regardless of whose name is on the asset. The combined assets a couple may retain and still qualify for Medicaid coverage of the nursing facility spouse are:

- the home in which the at-home spouse lives, regardless of its value;

- a Community Spouse Resource Amount equal to one-half the value of the couple's non-exempt liquid assets (such as cash, bank accounts, bonds) for the at-home spouse to use, in an amount of at least $16,000 but no more than $81,000; the maximum amount varies from state to state and both amounts increase yearly with the cost of living;

- one automobile, regardless of its value;

- furniture and household goods, regardless of value;

- one wedding and engagement ring each, regardless of value;

- life insurance with face value (the amount it would bring if cashed in) of $1,500;

- two burial plots and a separate savings account of up to $1,500 for each person for burial costs.

It is important to establish the total value of your assets through bank records or other documentation when the nursing facility spouse enters a nursing facility so that you can claim and retain one-half the full value.

MEDICAID WILL SEEK REIMBURSEMENT

A Medicaid recipient and his or her spouse may retain a certain amount of assets—including a home of any value if at least one of them lives in it—while Medicaid pays for long-term care. However, Medicaid has a right to seek reimbursement from the property of the Medicaid recipient for all Medicaid has spent on long-term care after the recipient turns age 55.

Medicaid cannot force the sale of a home while either spouse, or a minor or disabled child, lives in it. But it can seek reimbursement from the estate of the Medicaid recipient once the recipient and his or her spouse have both died. Those who take title to the property after the second spouse's death must either pay off the Medicaid amount or sell the property and have Medicaid collect its reimbursement out of the proceeds of the sale.

However, with some advance planning, it may be possible to protect the value of the property from some of Medicaid's reimbursement right. (See Chapter 7.)

B. What Medicaid Pays For

As with eligibility, what Medicaid covers and how much it pays varies by state. In general, though, Medicaid pays for extensive home care and the full cost of nursing facility care as long as either is necessary.

1. Medicaid-Certified Providers Only

Medicaid pays only for covered services performed by a Medicaid-certified provider. Some agencies and facilities do not meet Medicaid quality standards and therefore are not certified to participate in the program. Also, because Medicaid pays less than what agencies or facilities charge private consumers, some providers choose not to participate in the Medicaid program. However, some facilities will accept only private paying residents but permit a resident to remain after he or she has switched to Medicaid coverage. And some home care providers either do not meet Medicaid standards or choose not to participate because of Medicaid paperwork or wanting to be paid in cash.

It is important to find out whether a provider participates in Medicaid before you obtain service from it. This is particularly true for nursing facility residence. Even if you are not initially dependent on Medicaid, find out the facility's policy on Medicaid patients. Some facilities maintain different, less desirable rooms for Medicaid patients. Switching to Medicaid later may affect the quality of care you receive.

2. Medicaid Home Care Coverage

Unlike Medicare, Medicaid does not usually have stringent rules about either the kind or duration of home care services it covers. In most states, Medicaid pays most of a certified home care agency's reasonable costs, even if care is primarily custodial, and covers many services by non-agency providers, as long as they are Medicaid-certified. In some states, Medicaid also pays for extra-duty nursing, rehabilitation therapies provided outside the home, prescribed medications and medical supplies. To find out whether Medicaid covers a particular service in your state, check with both the provider of the service and your local social service office.

If Medicaid covers a service and the provider accepts payment from Medicaid, the provider cannot then charge you for any amounts over that payment. But, of course, the provider can and will charge you for services not covered by Medicaid.

In some states, Medicaid charges additional fees as noted below.

- **Enrollment Fee.** Some states charge a small, one-time only fee of a few dollars when you first enroll in Medicaid.
- **Monthly Premium.** States are allowed to charge a small fee to "medically needy" Medicaid participants—those who would not normally qualify because of their income or assets, but who become eligible because paying their medical bills would drop their income or assets below the eligibility levels. The amounts of these premiums vary but are usually only two or three dollars a month.
- **Co-payments.** States may charge a co-payment—as Medicare does for the first few days of nursing facility care—which is a fixed amount for each covered service you receive. This may be charged only to those who qualify for Medicaid as "medically needy" (see above) or to any Medicaid recipient of services the state Medicaid program is not required by federal law to cover, but which it covers anyway as an "optional" service.

3. Medicaid Nursing Facility Coverage

Unlike Medicare, Medicaid can be a lifesaver when it comes to nursing facility bills. In general, Medicaid pays for all levels of care in certified facilities for an indefinite period of time.

Levels of Care Covered

Medicaid in all states covers residence in certified skilled nursing facilities. But unlike Medicare, coverage does not require a prior hospital stay.

The greatest advantage Medicaid has over Medicare coverage is that state Medicaid programs also cover residence in certified intermediate care and custodial care facilities, as well as some assisted living residences in a few states. This means that Medicaid coverage exists for the situation that most commonly exhausts a family's savings: a long-term stay in a personal care facility where the resident receives primarily non-medical custodial care.

Unlike Medicare, Medicaid coverage is not limited to a certain number of days. Medicaid covers nursing facility residence indefinitely, although it will frequently review the level of care being received and may require that residence be shifted to a lower-level care facility if it determines a higher level of care is no longer medically necessary.

FACILITY MUST KEEP YOU IF YOU BEGIN MEDICAID COVERAGE

Many people enter a nursing facility as a privately paying resident, but later run out of money and become eligible for Medicaid. Since Medicaid does not pay as much as residents who pay privately, a nursing facility might prefer to move out someone who becomes eligible for Medicaid and move in a waiting resident who is able to pay on his or her own. But federal law forbids that.

Facilities that participate in the Medicaid program may not discharge a resident who becomes eligible for Medicaid. And as of 1999, a facility may not avoid this law even by withdrawing from the Medicaid program altogether. No one who resided in a facility while the facility participated in the Medicaid program may be discharged if he or she later becomes eligible for Medicaid, even if the facility drops out of the Medicaid program.

The only people left out of these legal protections are residents of facilities that have never participated in Medicaid, or who moved into a facility after it had already entirely dropped out of the Medicaid program.

How Much Medicaid Pays

Some state Medicaid programs pay only a certain percentage of the cost of care. Check in advance with both the facility and your local Medicaid social worker to determine what Medicaid will cover and how much it will pay.

In general, Medicaid pays a nursing or other qualifying residential facility a daily rate that covers medical and personal or custodial care, rehabilitation therapies provided by the facility, and room and board. And for whatever Medicaid covers, the facility must accept Medicaid's payment as payment in full. The facility cannot bill you for any additional amounts for covered services. Among the personal care items for which the facility may not charge extra to a Medicaid resident are: non-prescription drugs, incontinence supplies, razors, soaps and tooth care items and services such as laundry and basic hair and nail grooming. In some states, more items and services are covered. You can get a full list of what is covered from the facility, the facility's ombudsman or the social services office that administers Medicaid in the county in which the facility is located.

C. Finding Out About Medicaid in Your State

REMINDER

Before you apply for Medicaid, read Chapter 7 and consider taking the steps explained there that could help protect some of your assets from nursing facility and other costs.

To qualify for Medicaid, you must file a written application to the agency that handles Medicaid on the local level, usually the county

Department of Social Services, Health Department or Welfare Department. If you or a family member are already hospitalized or in a nursing facility, ask to have the medical social worker assist you in obtaining and filling out the applications.

There are a number of documents you should bring with you when you apply, most of which have to do with your financial situation. Even if you do not have the following documents, go ahead and begin the application process. The Medicaid eligibility workers can help you get whatever papers and documents are necessary, including:

- most recent interest and dividend statements, previous year's income tax return, recent pension and Social Security benefit papers or deposit slips indicating your current income;
- papers showing all your financial assets, such as bank books, insurance policies, stock certificates and car registration. If you used the assets worksheet in Chapter 1, bring documents reflecting all the assets you listed there;
- rent receipts, lease agreement or canceled rent checks if you are a renter, or mortgage payment book and latest tax assessment on the property if you're a home owner;
- your Social Security card or number;
- if you live with your spouse, information about his or her income and separate assets; and
- medical bills from the previous three months. And if you are planning on home care or residence in a care facility in the near future, bring medical records or reports that confirm your condition will require the particular care. If you don't have records or reports, bring the names and addresses of doctors who are treating you.

You will be interviewed and assisted in filling out your application by a Medicaid eligibility worker. Write down his or her name and telephone extension in case you have specific questions during the application process.

It may take several visits and there may be delays in processing your application while the proper documents are located and reviewed. Normally you will receive a decision within a few weeks; the law says a decision must be made within 45 days after your application is complete. If you don't hear from Medicaid within 30 days after completing your application, call the Medicaid social worker who interviewed you and ask what's going on. Social service and Medicaid agencies are very overworked and sometimes a person's application gets delayed in the shuffle. Stay on top of things so your application isn't delayed any more than necessary.

THE RETROACTIVE COVERAGE RULE

A valuable rule says that if you become eligible for Medicaid, you may be covered for home care or nursing facility costs back to the beginning of the third month before you filed your application. You must present proof of covered costs during that time. Make sure when you apply that your Medicaid eligibility worker knows you want retroactive coverage.

D. What to Do If You Are Denied Medicaid Coverage

If you are notified that you do not qualify for Medicaid, or that coverage is denied for a particular service, facility or time period, you have a right to what is called a "fair hearing" to determine if the decision is correct. If you receive notice of a decision you do not agree with, inquire immediately, at the office where you applied, about the procedure in your state for getting a fair hearing.

The rules for a fair hearing vary, but in general you are permitted to have a friend, relative, social worker, lawyer or other representative appear with you and testify about your financial situation, medical condition or expenses if such evidence would be helpful. The hearing itself is informal and you will be able to explain your position in your own words, without having to worry about legal technicalities or jargon. If your medical condition or need for treatment is the crucial question, a detailed letter from your doctor would be of great help. The hearing officer who makes the decision is not a judge but is a Medicaid eligibility specialist.

Although the odds of getting a Medicaid denial reversed at a fair hearing are not in your favor, such reversals do happen frequently enough, and the amount of money involved is large enough, that it is worth the effort. And even if the fair hearing officer decides against you, there may be procedures in your state for further appeal. Information about that appeal will probably be given to you along with the fair hearing decision. If not, check with your local social service office.

FREE ASSISTANCE GETTING NURSING FACILITY COVERAGE

If you are entering a nursing or personal care facility and are having trouble either being accepted for Medicaid or getting Medicaid to cover that facility, contact your state's Nursing Home Ombudsman. The ombudsman program is financed by the federal government and its purpose is to assist people with problems relating to nursing facilities. There is no charge for using its services. You can find your local office of the Nursing Home Ombudsman under that name in the white pages of your telephone directory, or through Senior Information and Referral. You can also be referred to the ombudsman through your area, state or local Agency on Aging, or through the central ombudsman office for your state. (See the Resource Directory in the Appendix at the back of this book.) ■

Medicaid and Asset Protection

A. Medicaid Rules on Transfer of Assets

As discussed in Chapter 6, a person is only eligible for Medicaid when his or her assets are reduced to minimum levels, which vary from state to state, with marital status, and from home care to residential facility. A person (and spouse) must personally pay all long-term care costs—home care, or nursing facility—until assets have been spent down to Medicaid levels.

To avoid spending all their savings on long-term care before Medicaid begins coverage, many people used to give away assets—or at least transfer legal title—to children or other relatives, then apply for Medicaid. But Medicaid rules now severely restrict such transfers. Today, there is no simple way to keep your assets and also qualify for Medicaid. Long-range planning may permit someone to qualify for Medicaid while his or her assets remain with family members, but only if personal control over the assets has been relinquished.

Before learning about the few ways by which some long-range planning can protect family assets, it is important to learn the basic rules by which Medicaid judges whether a transfer of one type of asset or another is proper.

1. Penalized Transfers

There is one basic Medicaid rule limiting the transfer of assets by nursing facility residents: Anything transferred from your name during the 36 months before either applying for Medicaid, or entering a nursing facility if you are already receiving Medicaid, is considered an invalid transfer. If the asset has not actually been transferred to another person, but has been placed in an irrevocable trust, the look back period is 60 months, not 36. The effect of this invalid transfer rule is that your eligibility for Medicaid is delayed for a period of time beginning on the date of transfer determined by the value of the asset transferred, divided by the average monthly nursing facility cost in your state.

Example. *You transfer a certificate of deposit worth $10,000 to your daughter a month before applying for Medicaid nursing facility coverage. The average monthly nursing facility cost in your state is $3,333. The penalty for your transfer within the 36-month period is figured by dividing the amount transferred ($10,000) by the average monthly nursing facility cost ($3,333), which equals 3. So, for three months from the date of the transfer, you would be ineligible for Medicaid and would have to pay your nursing facility costs yourself.*

A QUESTION OF ETHICS

The following section of this book discusses ways in which Medicaid rules permit people with assets that would make them ineligible for Medicaid coverage can transfer those assets to make them eligible, and for people to protect assets from Medicaid reimbursement. In other words, these rules permit people to keep their money and yet have their long-term care costs paid for by the government as if they had no money.

The rules and how some choose to apply them have rankled many. Medicaid was enacted as a safety net for the poor. Many elderly people truly become impoverished by a combination of high medical costs and low incomes. Medicaid saves their dignity, and prolongs their lives, by guaranteeing a decent level of care. But this care comes at a cost to taxpayers—a cost that our society has declared a willingness to pay. There has been no such public declaration, however, about the elderly who have assets. A truly compassionate society might provide free long-term care for all its citizens, but ours has not shown a willingness to pay—to be taxed—for it.

Despite recent closing of loopholes, some people with sizable assets are still able to skirt around the edges of the law and have Medicaid pick up the tab for their long-term care. Following the rules carefully makes this legal. Whether it is entirely ethical—that is, whether it is a violation of the spirit of the Medicaid law and of the position of those who have refused to support long-term care for all—is a different question. And one which each person who considers these rules must answer privately.

2. Permissible Transfers

Medicaid permits some exceptions to this 36-month rule. These exceptions are considerably different for an unmarried person and for a married couple. And they vary greatly between exempt and non-exempt assets. (To review which assets are exempt, review Chapter 6, Sections A1 and A2.)

The following assets may be transferred without incurring any eligibility penalty.

Unmarried Individuals

An unmarried person can transfer the assets listed below without any eligibility penalty.

Home. A home can be transferred:

- to the Medicaid applicant's minor child (through a custodianship or trust arrangement), or to the applicant's blind or disabled child of any age;
- to the applicant's child of any age who has lived in the home for two years prior to the parent's entry into a nursing facility and who cared for the parent, allowing the parent to remain at home rather than enter a nursing facility during that time;
- to a brother or sister who already has some ownership interest in the property and who has lived in the home for at least the previous year.

Other exempt assets. You may transfer to anyone, at any time, your car worth up to $4,500, personal or household belongings worth up to $2,000, your engagement or wedding rings, or other exempt assets. (See the list of exempt assets in Chapter 6.)

Non-exempt assets. You may transfer any asset, at any time, to your minor, blind or disabled child. You may also transfer any asset at any time to any person if you can prove to Medicaid that the purpose of the transfer was something *other* than to qualify for Medicaid, such as to help a relative in need.

Married People Entering a Nursing Facility

As discussed in Chapter 6, Section A, Medicaid rules give married couples an advantage over unmarried people in permitting an at-home spouse to retain some liquid assets and income. The rules also permit some additional benefit by allowing the couple to change the title on their home when one spouse enters a nursing facility.

Home. A married person can transfer title to a home to his or her spouse either before or after entering a nursing facility. Although the home is exempt anyway as long as the spouse is living in it, as is discussed more fully later in this chapter, it may be best to transfer title to the at-home spouse, who can then transfer the home to children or others in case the at-home spouse should die first. A married person can also transfer title to the home to any of the other people an unmarried person can transfer to, as described above.

Other exempt assets. A married person at any time can transfer exempt assets to anyone. (Refer to Chapter 6 for the list of a married couple's exempt assets.)

Other assets. You can transfer any assets, at any time, to your minor, blind or disabled child. Any asset can also be transferred to anyone at any time if it can be proved by the person transferring that the transfer was for some purpose other than to qualify for Medicaid. Such proof is difficult, however, and would require convincing testimony as to the validity of the reason for the transfer—for example, to help a brother or sister keep a failing business, or to pay a child's uninsured medical costs.

Before applying for Medicaid, a spouse may transfer any non-exempt asset to his or her at-home spouse, but only if the at-home spouse does not transfer it to anyone else within 36 months, for less than its true value. For example, title to non-exempt assets cannot be transferred to the sole name of the at-home spouse and then given immediately to the children.

B. Removing Assets From Medicaid Consideration

This section discusses two separate but related questions.

Transfers for eligibility. First, if you have too many assets to qualify for Medicaid, are there lawful ways to transfer some of those assets so that you become eligible for Medicaid?

Transfers for asset protection. Second, if you can qualify for Medicaid, are there lawful ways to transfer some assets so that they are out of reach when Medicaid seeks reimbursement after your death?

Each of the options discussed in this section has some drawbacks, and not all of them will be available to everyone. Carefully read through the rules to decide whether any of these options might be right for you.

1. Transfers 36 Months Before Medicaid Application

Although many people need long-term care as the result of an accidental injury or the sudden onset of illness—a stroke, heart attack— many others need care because of a slowly deteriorating physical or mental condition. If you are gradually heading toward the need for long-term care, one of the ways you may financially plan for it is to divest yourself of assets that might make you ineligible for Medicaid. Any asset transferred more than 36 months prior to applying for Medicaid is not considered in determining eligibility.

Along with the other methods described here, you may be able to transfer liquid assets to children or others who are the very people you would eventually want to get them. For many, the main problem with this approach is that when you give away assets, you lose control over them. If you later need the funds, or change your mind about giving them away, you must depend on the cooperation of those to whom you gave the assets. And you risk the possibility that they will no longer have them.

TAX CONSEQUENCES OF PROPERTY TRANSFERS

Transferring your home or other valuable assets may have unforeseen gift tax and income tax consequences. In general, an individual can make a gift valued up to $10,000 to another individual each year without any gift tax consequences. For example, if there are six people to whom you wish to make gifts (four adult children and two spouses of those children) you could make gifts totaling $60,000 per year. In addition, there is no gift tax for any amounts left to someone at death but given away to that person during one's lifetime if the total estate at death is valued under $600,000.

Income tax consequences have to do with the tax basis of the property, which is usually lower if property is given away upon death.

See Chapter 9 for a more detailed discussion of tax basis rules.

---

2. Investments in Your Home

Because Medicaid rules often exempt a home of any value from asset eligibility limits, concentrating your assets in your home is a good way to protect them. Investing in your home may help you qualify for Medicaid. And if you follow this type of investment with other steps discussed here, you may also protect the value added to your home from Medicaid claims for reimbursement. This is useful for both unmarried individuals and for couples, but the rules are different for each and must be carefully followed. Assuming you don't have other immediate needs for your savings or investments, you could put those assets into your home by:

- paying off your outstanding mortgage;
- making home improvements or large-scale repairs; or by

■ buying a new home or condominium for more money than your present home is worth. For the home to be protected, though, you or your spouse must live in it.

Home Investment by Unmarried Individuals

The ways in which an unmarried individual can invest in a home to affect Medicaid eligibility and reimbursement depend on whether the person remains living there or moves into a nursing facility. In either case, you may require some assistance from a lawyer or tax accountant familiar with Medicaid procedures. A brief explanation of the possible transfers follows.

Long-term home care. As long as an unmarried individual remains living at home, Medicaid will pay for long-term home care regardless of the value of the house. So, if a person has too many non-exempt assets to qualify for Medicaid, investing the excess assets in the house—which is not considered a transfer to anyone else—would permit the individual to qualify.

States without a strict "return home" rule. Medicaid rules in some states permit unmarried nursing facility residents to exempt their homes—meaning the value of their homes do not disqualify them from Medicaid coverage. This is true in these states even though there is little likelihood the individuals will return to live in those homes. The only requirement is that the individual entering a nursing facility must state on the admission form that he or she intends to return home. If you live in a state with such a rule, you may be free to invest assets in your home, making them exempt. Check with the local Department of Social Services, Health Department or Welfare Department to find out the current rule in your locale.

Exempt child or sibling. If your adult child or brother or sister lives in your home and would qualify the home as an exempt asset, you may want to invest further in the home. (See the explanation, above.)

Transfer to non-exempt adult child. Even if it would not qualify the house as an exempt asset, you may still want to consider investing assets in the house and transferring title to a son or daughter. This means giving up control over the property, so you must trust your child to manage it according to your wishes. Also, you must want the home to remain that child's property after your death.

The benefit of transferring your home to your child comes from not having to sell the home to pay your own nursing facility bills. If you transfer the home more than 36 months before you apply for Medicaid or enter a nursing facility, the value of the home will not affect your Medicaid eligibility at all. If you transfer it within 36 months before entering a nursing facility, your eligibility will be delayed for a period equal to the value of the home divided by the average monthly nursing facility cost in your state. (See the explanation of the Medicaid 36-month rule in Section A1 of this chapter.) For example, if the equity in your home is $100,000, you could be denied Medicaid coverage for 18 months to two years, depending on the cost of care in your state. One month of coverage is denied for roughly every $3,000 to $3,500 of equity.

Creating a life estate. A "life estate" is a legal maneuver that transfers title to property, without affecting who has use of the property.

Here's how it works. A legal document is drawn up creating a life estate in the home, which permits the elder to live there for the rest of his or her life. The life estate "remainder"—the value remaining after the death of the homeowner—goes to the homeowner's children, or any other person designated, upon the homeowner's death.

The Medicaid advantage of a life estate is that in calculating an unmarried person's assets, most states normally count the full value of the home. The homeowner must sell it and use the funds to pay for nursing facility care before becoming eligible for Medicaid. With a life estate, the elder no longer has the value of the home as an asset, but only has the value of remaining there for life. If a person must enter a nursing facility with the possibility of not returning home, and if returning, of not living many years there, then the value of the life estate is far smaller than the value of the home. The elder would only be required to spend an amount equal to the value of the life estate, rather than the greater value of the home, before being eligible for Medicaid.

Creating a life estate for Medicaid purposes is a technical legal maneuver that requires sound advice and assistance from an attorney experienced in estate planning and Medicaid rules.

Home Investment by Couples

A home is a particularly good place for a married couple to invest savings or other assets. Even if one spouse enters a nursing facility, as long as the other spouse lives at home, it is completely exempt from Medicaid eligibility limits no matter how much it is worth.

Investing in the home may only be the beginning of protecting assets there. You can take additional steps to further protect those assets:

Title transfer to spouse. If one spouse enters a nursing facility, he or she should transfer sole title to the property to the spouse who remains at home. The spouse at home should then transfer the property to children or anyone else other than the nursing facility spouse. The transfer can be by immediate gift, or through a provision in a will or living trust under which the property will not actually transfer until the at-home spouse's death.

This transfer avoids the consequences that would occur if the nursing facility spouse's name remained on title to the property, but the at-home spouse died first. In that case, the value of the home would be used to reimburse Medicaid for all the money it had spent on care for the nursing facility spouse.

Also, once the home is in the sole name of the at-home spouse, he or she may be able to make good use of its equity, for example, by selling the home and using the money. There are also other equity conversion devices, such as reverse annuity mortgages in which a home with a large amount of equity is used as collateral for a loan and the lender makes monthly or lump sum payments to the homeowner. One such method might provide income, some of which could be protected from Medicaid consideration.

To know what transfer of title, sale of your home, living trusts or equity conversion devices might mean for you in terms of tax advantages and disadvantages measured against Medicaid eligibility, it is recommended that you seek the advice of a lawyer, accountant, or business adviser who is familiar with both Medicaid rules and tax laws.

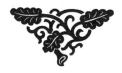

MEDICAID MAY RECOVER COST OF CARE

Medicaid has the right to collect the entire amount it has spent on long-term care—whether home care, community care or care in a nursing facility—for anyone age 55 or over. It does so out of any assets in the Medicaid recipient's estate at death. If assets have been lawfully transferred out of the Medicaid recipient's name before death, and without violating Medicaid's transfer rules (see Section A2), then those assets would be out of reach for Medicaid reimbursement.

Usually, the largest asset from which Medicaid can seek reimbursement is the recipient's home. Medicaid can place a lien on the property and collect on the lien whenever the property is sold, if the recipient:

- is in a nursing facility,
- is not expected to return home as certified by a physician, and
- has no spouse, minor or disabled child or sibling with an equity interest in the property living in the home.

However, if the recipient, spouse or minor or disabled child or sibling with an equity interest in the property is living in the home, or the recipient intends to return to the home, the rule is different. In these situations, Medicaid cannot place a lien on the home but must wait to collect its reimbursement out of the recipient.

The amount Medicaid is entitled to be reimbursed may be decreased if the Medicaid recipient had secured a state partnership long-term care insurance policy. (See Section B8.)

3. Investing in Other Exempt Assets

A home is not the only asset automatically exempt from Medicaid eligibility limits. Those listed below are also exempt, and up to each state's limits, can be invested in without affecting Medicaid eligibility:

- an automobile (up to $4,500 for an individual, of any value for a couple);
- furniture and household goods (up to $2,000 for an individual, of any value for a couple);
- one wedding and one engagement ring per person of any value (individual or couple). They don't have to be the original engagement or wedding rings—one can buy a new ring at any time, so it is possible to put some assets into valuable rings; and
- a burial plot and separate burial fund up to a value of $1,500.

4. Transferring Non-Exempt Assets to At-Home Spouse

Although transferring non-exempt assets from a nursing facility spouse to an at-home spouse will not initially protect those assets from being counted toward Medicaid eligibility limits (unless they are then transferred to others before Medicaid is applied for, see Section 1, above), such a transfer can save as much as $79,000 if the at-home spouse dies before the nursing facility spouse.

Example. *When one spouse is a resident in a nursing facility, Medicaid counts the joint assets of the couple and allows the couple to keep one-half of those combined assets—in some states up to $81,000. But an unmarried nursing facility resident can keep only about $2,000. If the at-home spouse dies, the spouse in the nursing facility becomes an unmarried individual who can only keep $2,000, and the $81,000 the couple had been allowed to keep then automatically goes to pay nursing facility bills.*

A couple can avoid losing most of this $80,000 by taking two simple steps. First, the nursing facility spouse transfers the $80,000 into the sole name of the at-home spouse. Then, the at-home spouse makes a will or creates a living trust that leaves the money to the children or to anyone other than the nursing facility spouse. If the at-home spouse dies first, the money goes to the children or other named beneficiary, and not to the nursing facility. (See next section.)

5. Transferring Assets to Children or Others

Some methods of protecting your assets by transferring them to your children or to anyone else other than your spouse, without jeopardizing your Medicaid nursing facility eligibility, have already been mentioned. Here are a couple more points to consider when transferring assets. Remember, though, that transferring assets to children or others means giving up control of those assets. If you need to use the assets, you must depend on the goodwill of your children or anyone else to whom you have transferred them.

Transfers of Exempt Assets

Specifically exempt assets—home, car, household goods—may be transferred to children or anyone else even within the 36-month Medicaid no-transfer period. But if assets are exempt, why bother to transfer them? Look back at the Medicaid rules for exempt assets (Chapter 6) and you will see that the exemptions for a married couple with one spouse in a nursing facility are far more generous than for an unmarried individual. But if the at-home spouse dies, a couple's exempt property—home, up to $80,000 in savings, car and household goods of any value—instantly becomes an unmarried person's non-exempt property, and so a source for nursing facility bills. To protect against that, some people transfer title to exempt property as well.

6. Payments to Children for Services

Unmarried individuals are at a disadvantage in trying to pass assets to their children or others. Because there is no spouse through whom assets can be transferred, many Medicaid exemption rules do not apply. One way around the 36-month transfer rule is not to transfer assets at all, but instead to pay a child or other person for services performed for you. Such services might be personal care or assistance, transportation, housekeeping, paperwork—almost any reasonable service you would otherwise have to pay someone else to do. Because these are payments rather than transfers, they do not count as transferred assets. However, the Internal Revenue Service and state tax agencies consider these payments as income to the people receiving them, and may require payment of income tax on the amounts received.

As you might guess, Medicaid looks very closely at such arrangements. The services performed must be reasonable and there must be proof they were actually performed. Also, the payments must be reasonable for the services rendered: a thousand dollars for one housecleaning won't pass muster. But payment to an adult child or grandchild for regular housecleaning and maintenance, or for regular transportation, for example, might be acceptable if the amounts paid are within range of the amounts which would have to be paid to a private housecleaning service or for a taxi.

7. Medicaid and Divorce

It may seem strange to think of divorce in connection with long-term care, but the unfortunate effect of the Medicaid income and assets limits has been to force more than a few couples to divorce for solely economic reasons. If all other methods for transferring or otherwise protecting assets are unavailable, or the eligibility problem is with continuing income, you may at least want to consider the unpleasant alternative of divorce. Remember, though, that all that is required to change Medicaid status is the formal, legal divorce. A couple need not stop living together, but they must separate their bank accounts and joint income, change title to property and otherwise shift their financial interests to reflect separate lives. Any asset they continue to own or control jointly will be considered part of the Medicaid applicant's assets.

This situation often arises when a couple must choose between entering a nursing facility and being covered by Medicaid, or remaining home without coverage. About thirty states have no income eligibility levels for Medicaid coverage of residential nursing facility care; the other states have income levels of $700 to $1,100 per month for eligibility, but allow the at-home spouse to keep all income in his or her name. And all states allow the at-home spouse of a nursing facility resident to keep between $12,000 and $80,000 in savings or other assets.

For non-nursing facility care, on the other hand, all states have severe limits on the amount of income and assets a couple can have and still qualify for Medicaid coverage. A couple may thus be forced to choose between getting care at home and being disqualified from Medicare, or getting divorced. A divorce permits the working spouse to keep all of his or her income without disqualifying the other spouse and allows the protection of at least half of the couple's assets without limit. The spouse (now ex-spouse) needing care can then remain at home and receive Medicaid-covered home care.

A couple may face the same difficult choice about whether to end their marriage for economic reasons even when one spouse is already in a nursing facility. If they live in a state with income eligibility limits for nursing facility couples and the at-home spouse continues to work and make more than the allowable income, that would disqualify the nursing facility spouse from coverage. Similarly, if a couple has considerably more in savings and other non-exempt assets than the Medicaid rules of their state would permit them to keep, a divorce settlement that gives more assets to the at-home spouse than Medicaid would have allowed the couple to keep may be a way of holding on to savings.

These are all matters that depend, however, on both the specific Medicaid rules and divorce laws of your state. If divorce seems like the best last resort for you, consult a lawyer who is familiar both with divorce law and with Medicaid.

8. Special Insurance Available in Some States

Programs in California, Connecticut, Indiana and New York provide some asset protection through the purchase of special long-term care insurance policies. These states have watched many people use asset transfers to spend down their assets and then qualify for Medicaid— costing their state programs huge amounts of money. To get more people with assets and income to pay for some of their own long-term care, the Medicaid programs in these states encourage people to buy special state-certified long-term care insurance policies to cover a portion of their care. In exchange for people buying the insurance, Medicaid promises to permit the insured person to keep more assets than normal Medicaid rules permit.

There are two types of these programs, and they protect different amounts of assets in different ways.

California, Connecticut and Indiana

In the California, Connecticut and Indiana programs, the amount of assets protected above each state's normal asset limits equals the amount of benefits paid under the special long-term care insurance policy. In other words, when the insured person applies for Medicaid coverage, whatever the special insurance policy has paid out in benefits is added to the amount of assets the Medicaid applicant is entitled to keep. These state partnership policies must also offer some home care benefits, some automatic inflation protection and a non-forfeiture benefit.

Example. *Mr. X purchased a state partnership long-term care policy. The policy paid $100 per day in nursing facility costs for Mr. X for two years, for a total of $73,000. Mr. X qualified for Medicaid coverage for continuing long-term care after his insurance benefits ran out and as soon as his savings and other countable assets were down to $73,000. Without the policy, Mr. X would have had to spend his savings down to $2,000 before Medicaid would have started to pay for his long-term care costs.*

New York

The New York model goes even farther in protecting assets and in specifying the policy terms to be offered.

Policy terms. The New York partnership policies cover at least $100 per day in a nursing facility for three years and $50 per day home care for six years. The premiums for this coverage run about $1,000 per year if purchased at age 55, about $2,500 per year at age 70.

Medicaid payments. When the insurance policy benefits run out and the insured still requires long-term care, Medicaid will then pay part of long-term care costs. The insured person must still pay part of costs out of any income he or she has, including Social Security. The insured is only allowed to keep $525 per month income if living at home, $50 per month if living in a nursing facility.

Asset protection. The insured person can collect Medicaid and still retain all of his or her assets, no matter how great. As indicated above, however, income is not protected.

State Partnership Long-term Care Insurance

Additional benefits and risks

In addition to their asset-protecting terms, most policies offered under these state partnership programs also have other relatively good features. They are required to offer—at some additional cost—home and community care coverage in addition to institutional care. Most of these policies offer good benefits, inflation protection and level premiums. (See Chapter 10 for an explanation of these terms and their importance in choosing a policy.)

But as with all long-term care insurance, if you are considering a state partnership policy, carefully compare all its terms with other policies. Although these Medicaid-partner policies have generally good terms and the advantage of some asset protection, for most consumers they also present the same basic risks as do other long-term care policies. The first and foremost of these risks is that, as explained in Chapter 10, any long-term care policy is a gamble. These partnership policies, like all others, are expensive. Over years, you pay significant premiums to protect against the chance that you will someday need long-term care for two, three or more years that would, without the insurance, surely eat up all your assets.

The probability of the need for a two-or three-year period of nursing facility care, however, is only about 30% for women and 15% for men who reach age 65. Of those people, only about 10% to 15% remain in a nursing facility for more than three years. The numbers of people who need some sort of long-term home care is greater, but the average cost of such care is significantly less than for institutional care. If it turns out that you do not need long-term care at all, or need it only for a relatively short time, all the money you spend on years of insurance premiums will have been wasted.

A second risk is the possibility that at some point you will be unable to afford to continue paying premiums and therefore will lose your coverage. Even state partnership policies are expensive, and if your income drops in your later years, the premiums may become too much for your budget. If so, you may decide you have to drop your coverage just when you are coming up to the years when you are most likely to need it. And the years of premiums you have already paid would wind up being nearly a total loss, depending on the level of reduced benefits or the non-forfeiture provision in your policy. (See Chapter 10, Section G.)

Another risk with an asset-protecting policy is that the cost of long-term care in some urban areas may eat up most of your assets before Medicaid ever kicks in to cover you. For example, if you have a policy that pays $100 per day in nursing facility costs, but the facility you choose charges $175 per day—as many do in California, Connecticut and New York—the uncovered part of your costs ($75/day) would mount up to $82,000 in three years. So, if you have well over $100,000 in assets to protect in addition to your home, the policy might work to preserve a portion of those assets. If you have less than $100,000 in assets other than your home, the policy would allow you to save very little even though you have spent a tremendous amount in premiums over the years.

For some people, a major drawback with these asset-protection policies is that they do not protect income. If you expect to continue having substantial income while you receive long-term care, that income will be unprotected and may disqualify you from Medicaid even though your assets would otherwise be protected. Only a very small amount of income—$50 to $75 per month for a nursing facility resident; $500 to $600 per month for a home care recipient—is protected under these policies.

A major risk factor with these state partnership policies is that if you wind up receiving care in another state, that other state's Medicaid program will not honor the agreement with the state where you bought the policy. The policy itself will remain enforceable—the insurance company must pay benefits—but the asset-protection provision will have gone out the window because you will be bound by the new state's Medicaid rules. This problem may present a particular risk if you are in your 50s or 60s when you buy a policy, since it may be uncertain that you will remain in the same state for the next 20 to 30 years. It may also be risky if most or all of your supporting family—siblings, children, adult grandchildren—live in other states. If so, when you do need care, it is likely you will want to receive it near family.

Finally, all the other pitfalls of long-term care insurance apply to Medicaid partner policies as well. These problems are discussed in Chapter 10. Before buying any long-term care policy, read that chapter carefully and examine and compare all the terms of an asset-protecting policy just as you would any other long-term care policy.

■

Protecting Choices About Medical Care and Finances

One of the difficult truths of aging is that when physical or mental capacities diminish, many elders must depend on others to take care of life's business for them. A number of legal and practical roadblocks often complicate this shifting of responsibilities, however. And if an elder becomes entirely incapable of making decisions, there can be enormous problems, not only in getting matters decided, but in deciding them as the elder would wish.

This chapter discusses how elders can ensure that their rights, dignity and wishes are protected if they were to become incapable of making or communicating decisions about medical interventions. It also discusses how elders can prepare to have their finances managed for them if they become incapable of doing so.

A. Health Care Decisions

The increasing use of life-sustaining medical technology over the last decades has raised fears in many of us that our lives may be artificially prolonged against our wishes. The right to die with dignity, and without the tremendous agony and expense for both patient and family caused by prolonging life artificially, has been addressed now by the U.S. Supreme Court, the federal government and every state.

And the right to control medical decisions also extends to situations where doctors might wish to provide a patient with less extensive care than he or she would like. For example, a doctor may be reluctant to administer long-term treatments to a patient who has slim chances of recovering.

In 1990, the United States Supreme Court held that every individual has the constitutional right to control his or her own medical treatment. The Court also declared that "clear and convincing evidence" of a person's wishes must be followed by medical personnel. (*Cruzan v. Director, Missouri Dept. of Health*, 497 U.S. 261.)

1. Documents Protecting Medical Care Choices

Every state now has laws authorizing individuals to create a health care directive—a simple document that provides the "clear and convincing evidence" of that person's wishes concerning life-prolonging medical care. Depending upon the state, the document may be called by one of several different names: Living Will or Declaration.

The directions expressed in the document are to be followed if an individual is no longer capable of communicating to medical personnel his or her choices regarding life-prolonging and other medical care. It is important to note that these documents take effect only when a patient is diagnosed to have a terminal condition, to be in a permanent coma or in a few states, diagnosed with some additional serious medical condition. Health care directives are not used when a person is able to communicate those wishes to doctors in any way or is only temporarily unconscious or incapacitated.

Your written medical care instructions can help alleviate your fears either that unwanted medical treatment will be administered to you or that desired medical treatment will be withheld. It can also help relieve family members from having to make agonizing decisions about your medical treatment. This can be particularly important when family members have conflicting ideas about what care you should receive. Also, doctors and hospitals have their own rules and beliefs about what is proper medical treatment, and even if your family knows your wishes and tries to have them followed, medical personnel would not necessarily be bound to follow them unless you have completed and signed a valid document.

2. Differences Among Medical Care Documents

The two basic types of document to direct medical care are a Living Will—also called Directive to Physicians or Declaration—and a Durable Power of Attorney for Health Care or Health Care Proxy.

The basic difference between the two types of document is simple. The Living Will, Directive or Declaration is a statement you make directly to medical personnel which spells out the medical care you do or do not wish to receive if you become terminally ill and incapacitated. It acts as a contract with the treating doctor, who must either honor the wishes for medical care that you have expressed—or transfer you to another doctor or facility that will honor them.

In a Durable Power of Attorney or Health Care Proxy, you can appoint someone else to oversee your doctors to make sure they provide you with the kind of medical care you wish to receive. In some states, you can also give the person you appoint the broader authority to make decisions about your medical care on your behalf. In some states, you may express both wishes for your medical care and name a person to oversee them in a single document.

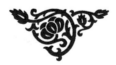

WHEN YOUR STATE FORM IS NOT ENOUGH

As mentioned, when it comes to medical directives, there are many state differences in the forms and formats used. Some state laws require that a specific form must be used for a directive to be valid. However, since the Supreme Court ruled in the *Cruzan* case that every individual has a constitutional right to direct his or her own medical care, the most important thing for you to keep in mind is that your directions should be clear to doctors and other medical personnel. If you feel strongly about a particular kind of care—even if your state law or the form you get does not mention it—it is a good idea to include your specific requests. If you are using a specific state form that does not adequately address your concerns, write them in on the form with the additional request that your wishes be respected and followed.

---

3. What to Include in a Medical Directive

In completing their state forms on directing health care, many people are unsure how to fill in the blanks—and are unsure what much of the terminology means. Although medical technology and treatments are evolving over time, filling out the forms is not as difficult as it may seem at first. In most health care documents, you can direct:

- that all life-prolonging procedures be provided;
- that all life-prolonging procedures be withheld; or
- that some be provided—particularly comfort care, as discussed below—while others are withheld.

The following medical procedures and treatments are usually considered to be in the category of "life-prolonging." You can include specific directions as to some or all of them.

- *Artificial breathing apparatus, such as a respirator or ventilator.* Some people specify that they wish artificial breathing while they are conscious, but not if they lapse into unconsciousness.
- *Artificial administration of food and water, also called nutrition and hydration.* As with artificial breathing, some people want artificial food and water administered as long as they are conscious, but not if they become unconscious. A few states, however, do not permit a doctor or hospital to withhold artificial food and water even if you request that it be withheld. Again, if you feel strongly that you would want artificial food and water withheld, but you live in a state that restricts your right to direct that, add your request to the health care directive you fill out—and ask that your wishes be respected and followed, as is your constitutional right.
- *Comfort care—including relief from pain and discomfort, usually through medication.* Many people specify that they do want pain medication, but do not want any other life-prolonging measures.

Making decisions about your medical care

To make an informed decision about which procedures you do and do not want, it may be a good idea to discuss your medical directive with your physician. He or she can explain the medical procedures more fully and can discuss the options with you. You will also find out whether your doctor has any medical or moral objections to following your wishes. If he or she does object and will not agree to follow your wishes, you may want to consider changing doctors.

Even when you have specified your wishes in a medical directive regarding life-prolonging and comfort care medical treatment, certain matters may still be difficult to resolve. They include:

- when, exactly, to administer or withhold certain medical treatments;

- whether or not to provide, withhold or continue antibiotic or pain medication; and
- whether to pursue complex, painful and expensive surgeries which may serve to prolong life but cannot reverse the medical condition.

To deal with these situations, in most states, the document called a Power of Attorney for Health Care or Health Care Proxy allows you to appoint someone who understands your wishes and whose judgment you trust to make these decisions in accordance with your wishes and in your best interest. To help the appointed person make and carry out these decisions, the power of attorney or proxy form may include specific authorizations:

- to give, withhold or withdraw consent to medical or surgical procedures;
- to consent to appropriate care for the end of life, including pain relief;
- to hire and fire medical personnel;
- to visit you in the hospital or other facility even when other visiting is restricted;
- to have access to medical records and other personal information; and
- to get any court authorization required to obtain or withhold medical treatment if, for any reason, a hospital or doctor does not honor the document.

4. Choosing a Health Care Attorney-in-Fact or Proxy

There are a number of things to consider in choosing a health care attorney-in-fact or proxy. Some are obvious: you should choose someone who understands your wishes and whom you trust to follow those wishes.

But there are a few other things you should also consider, such as appointing someone who:

- is likely to be present when decisions need to be made—most often, this means someone who lives nearby or who is willing to travel and spend time to be at your side during your hospitalization

- would not easily be bullied or intimidated by doctors or family members who disagree with your wishes, and

- is capable of understanding your medical condition and the proposed life-prolonging measures.

It is also a good idea to appoint a second person as a backup or replacement attorney-in-fact or proxy to act if your first choice is unable or unwilling to serve. Make it clear, however, that the second person is only a back-up. It is not wise to appoint co-proxies: two people who must make decisions would only complicate the process.

 DO NOT APPOINT YOUR DOCTOR

Although your doctor is an important person for your attorney-in-fact or proxy to consult concerning all health care decisions, you should not appoint your doctor to act as attorney-in-fact or proxy. The laws in most states specifically forbid treating physicians from acting in this role—to avoid the appearance that they may have their own interests at heart and so may not be able to act purely according to your wishes.

---

5. Changing Your Mind—and Documents

Any type of medical directive can be changed by the person who made it as long as he or she remains legally competent to do so. Therefore, neither your decisions about health care nor about the proxy you have named are necessarily final decisions. Anytime you wish to change the terms or the proxy, however, you must prepare a new document and date, sign and have it witnessed and possibly notarized again—depending on the formalities that must be followed in your state. You should also make sure that all copies of the document you made earlier are destroyed.

6. Legal Rules and Conditions

As mentioned, each state makes its own rules concerning medical directives. Here are some of the rules and conditions of which you should be aware.

Required form. In some states, the document you use must contain some language specifically required by special provisions in state law. (See Section 7, below.)

Signing, witnessing, notarizing. Every state law requires that you sign your documents—or direct another person to sign them for you—as a way of verifying that you understand them and that they contain your true wishes.

Most state laws also require that you sign your documents in the presence of witnesses. The purpose of this additional formality is so that at least one other person can attest that you were the person that signed the document, and that you were of sound mind and of legal age when you did so.

QUALIFICATIONS FOR WITNESSES

Many states require that two witnesses see you sign your health care documents and that they verify in writing that you appeared to be of sound mind and signed the documents without anyone else influencing your decision.

Each state's qualifications for these witnesses are slightly different. In many states, for example, a spouse, other close relative or any person who would inherit property from you is not allowed to act as a witness for the document directing health care. And many states prohibit your attending physician from being a witness. In others, the person named as attorney-in-fact or proxy cannot also serve as a witness to the document.

The purpose of the laws restricting who can witness your documents is to avoid any appearance or possibility that another person was acting against your wishes in encouraging specific medical choices. States that prevent close relatives or potential inheritors from being witnesses, for example, justify their restrictions by noting that these people may be specially influenced by another person's health care.

In addition to the requirement that witnesses sign your medical directives, some states also require that you and the witnesses appear before a notary public and swear that the circumstances of your signing, as described on the documents, are true. In some states, you have the option of having a notary sign your document instead of having it witnessed.

7. Obtaining the Right Medical Directive Form

Be advised that the laws on medical directives and forms approved for use frequently change, so a particular form which was the right one in your state several years ago may by now have been replaced by a different, more complete form.

In most instances, you do not need to consult a lawyer to prepare a Living Will, Directive to Physicians, Power of Attorney for Health Care or other medical directive form. The forms for use in your state are usually quite simple, can be completed without a lawyer's help and can be obtained, free or for a nominal fee, from a number of sources, such as:

Senior referral & information. The white pages in most telephone directories have a listing for Senior Referral & Information. This number refers people to various agencies, groups and other sources of assistance for seniors. Call your local Senior Referral & Information number and ask where you can obtain your state's official medical directive form.

Local senior center. Often, your local senior center will have copies of your state's form for medical directive. If it does not have a copy, it may be able to obtain one for you.

Consumer organization. The national non-profit organization Choice in Dying (formerly the Society for the Right to Die) is one of the nation's oldest patients' advocacy groups. It provides information on your state's current laws on medical directives.

Choice in Dying
1035 30th Street, NW
Washington, DC 20007
800-989-9455
Internet: http://www.choices.org

Computer program. Nolo has developed WillMaker, an easy-to-use software program that helps you prepare and update a medical directive for any state—as well as a regular legal will, durable power of attorney for finances (see Section B) and final arrangements such as body donation, cremation or burial and funeral wishes. It comes with a manual providing necessary background information, and leads you - tep-by-step through the process.

8. What to Do With Your Completed Documents

Once you have completed the documents directing your medical care, there are several additional steps you should take.

Making and distributing copies. Ideally, you should make an effort to make your wishes for your future health care widely known. Keep a copy of your health care directives, and give other copies to:

- any physician with whom you consult regularly;
- any attorney-in-fact or health care proxy you have named;
- the office of the hospital or other care facility in which you are likely to receive treatment;
- the patient representative of your HMO or insurance plan;
- close relatives, particularly immediate family members—a spouse, children, siblings;
- trusted friends; and
- clergy or lawyer, particularly if you are in regular contact with the clergy or lawyer but you do not have a family member who lives nearby.

Keeping your documents up-to-date. Review your health care documents occasionally—at least once a year—to make sure they still accurately reflect your wishes for your medical care. Advances in technology and changes in health care prompt many people to change their minds about the kind of medical care they want.

In addition, you should consider making new documents if:

- you move to another state;
- you made and finalized a health care directive, but did so many years ago, before there may have been substantial changes to your state's law controlling them; or

■ the proxy or representative you named to supervise your wishes becomes unable to do so or you wish to change your proxy or representative.

KEEPING TRACK OF COPIES

Keep a signed copy of your medical directive in an easily accessible place at home—someplace you could easily describe to someone else if they had to retrieve it for you.

Also, keep a list of all the people and places that have copies of your medical directive. Then, if you change the terms of the directive, you will be able to retrieve each of the old copies or have them destroyed.

B. Power of Attorney for Finances

Wills and probate can take care of the distribution of income and assets after a person dies, but they do not cover financial matters during a period of incapacity before death. And for many people, such a period of incapacity lasts months, even years. A document called a durable power of attorney for finances can fill that gap.

A durable power of attorney for finances can be used to ensure that your financial matters are handled as you wish. Because it is a "durable" power of attorney, it remains effective if you become incapacitated. If you prefer, you can make a "springing" document—that is, a durable power of attorney that takes effect only if you can no longer manage your own financial affairs.

A durable power of attorney for finances can provide some peace of mind that your money and property will be managed by a trusted person according to your wishes—and without the need for a guardianship or conservatorship, court procedures that can be cumbersome and expensive.

Your document can be tailored to your specific financial situation, authorizing the person you choose—called your attorney in-fact—to take care of financial matters ranging from buying holiday gifts and keeping a garden tended to paying bills, making bank deposits, handling insurance, Social Security and other paperwork—even selling a home or other property. And the durable power of attorney for finances can also ensure that there is someone to pay for needed pain relief, comfort care or other medical treatment which may not be fully covered by Medicare and health insurance.

The success of any power of attorney arrangement depends upon the trust and understanding between you and the person you appoint as your attorney-in-fact. This understanding and trust can be supported by specific instructions in the document regarding particular financial actions you do and do not wish the attorney-in-fact to take.

As with a durable power of attorney for health care, you can change the attorney-in-fact or other terms of the document at any time, as long as you are legally competent. (See Section A8 for advice on what to do with your completed durable power of attorney for finances document.)

POWERS OF ATTORNEY AND MEDICAID

As explained in Chapter 7, there are several ways to protect your assets from the reach of a nursing facility while still qualifying for Medicaid. Several of these methods, however, might require a transfer of assets after you are no longer capable of doing so. If you create a durable power of attorney for finances, you may want to include the power to transfer title of property and other assets to a spouse, children or other specifically named people—the same people to whom you would want the property to pass after your death.

C. Guardianships and Conservatorships

Much of the advice so far in this chapter may not apply to you if the elder you are concerned about is already incapacitated and unable to make decisions. At that point, the elder can no longer enter into legal documents and arrangements or delegate responsibility for decisions to others. Yet there is a danger that without prior legal arrangements such as a durable power of attorney, financial institutions, government agencies, health care providers and bureaucrats of every variety will either refuse to take action regarding the elder's affairs—or will take actions without regard for your wishes or for what you know are the elder's wishes.

In this situation, you may have to go to court to ask a judge to appoint you or another friend or relative to act on the elder's behalf. There are procedures in every state to do this. Some states have only one legal category, usually called guardianship, while others have a second category, usually called conservatorship and often limited to financial matters.

In general guardianship proceedings, the legal question is whether or not the elder has become "incompetent" to handle any of his or her own affairs. In about half the states, this requires that medical evidence of incompetence be presented to the court. In more limited proceedings to establish a financial conservatorship or guardianship only (see below), the court can act if it finds that the elder is unable to handle financial affairs even though not completely legally incompetent.

In conservatorship or guardianship proceedings, an elder has a right to appear in court with an attorney and to consent or object to all proposed authority. In many states, if the elder does not have an attorney, the court may appoint one. Similarly, any change in the conservator or guardian's authority requires an additional court order to which the elder can consent or object. The conservator or guardian is held responsible for mismanagement of the elder's property.

In some states, it is possible to handle conservatorship proceedings without the assistance of a lawyer if no one challenges the need for the conservatorship and its scope. More complicated guardianship procedures, however, do require the assistance of a lawyer, particularly if the elder or anyone else does not agree that the guardianship is needed or that the person seeking to be guardian is not the right person for the job.

1. Financial Conservatorship or Guardianship

A conservator or guardian can be appointed by a court solely to protect an elder's property—savings, real estate, investments. He or she can also conduct daily financial affairs, such as paying bills, or arrange for services when the elder is unable to do so. This type of limited management assistance is appropriate when the elder is still capable of caring for himself or herself, but because of disorientation or disability is unable to carry out personal business affairs efficiently. In this situation, the conservator or guardian does not have power over the elder's personal conduct, but has authority over financial or other affairs as the court orders.

An advantage of a limited conservatorship or guardianship is that it leaves an elder free to make many important decisions independently: where to live, with whom to associate, what medical care to receive, how to handle property. Nonetheless, it is still a court process in which a judge makes a ruling, occasionally against the elder's will, that gives another person authority over some parts of his or her life. It is therefore a procedure to be used only if no other solution seems feasible.

2. Full Guardianship

Full guardianship is an extreme measure that severely restricts the legal rights of an elder based on a court's finding of legal incompetence. It reduces one's legal status to that of a minor, with no control over one's own money or property, decisions about medical care or institutionalization. A person under guardianship even loses the right to vote.

If an elder retains some degree of orientation and capability, a legal finding by a court that he or she is incompetent can be emotionally devastating and, in fact, self-fulfilling. The person deemed legally incompetent may well give up the will to care for himself or herself and become much less competent than before. Obviously, full guardianship is a very serious step, to be taken when a person's mental condition leaves no other choice.

CONSERVATORSHIPS, GUARDIANSHIPS AND MEDICAID

A conservator or guardian is under a legal obligation to act only in the best interests of the elder. As has been discussed over the last three chapters, there are times when the best interests of the elder with respect to qualifying for Medicaid may involve transferring assets to a spouse, child or other person. Taken at face value, giving away someone's property does not appear to be in that person's best interests. Therefore, before a conservator or guardian transfers an elder's property for Medicaid purposes, it is advisable to go to court, explain the proposed transfer and get the court's approval. ■

Estate Planning: Controlling Your Money and Property

Estate planning refers to actions you can take while living to determine what happens to your property when you die. It can include:

- deciding who will get your property when you die;
- setting up procedures and devices to make sure your property passes to others free from probate, or that your estate owes the least amount possible in probate fees;
- particularly if your estate is a large one, setting up ways to pass your property to others while reducing or avoiding taxes; and
- setting up management for property you want to go to others who might need outside help in managing it—including minors, an older or unhealthy spouse or companion or a person with tendencies to being a spendthrift or substance abuser.

Some people leave estate planning to lawyers, although the basic steps are easy enough to do yourself if you are willing to spend some time wading through rules and making some difficult decisions. The discussion in this chapter is by no means a comprehensive guide to estate planning, but it should help alert you to some of your options.

ESTATE PLANNING RESOURCES FROM NOLO

Nolo publishes many resources that can help you with estate planning. You may conclude that our recommendation is a little prejudiced, but we believe these are the best books and software available. And we offer a money-back guarantee if you do not agree. See the catalog at the back of this book for more information. Or visit our website at: http://www.nolo.com.

Books

- *The Conservatorship Book* (California only). Guidance for determining when a conservatorship is necessary for a person incapacitated due to illness or age and a discussion of possible alternatives.

- *8 Ways to Avoid Probate*. A guide to eight easy and inexpensive methods of transferring assets without going through probate.

- *The Financial Power of Attorney Workbook: Who Will Handle Your Finances If You Can't?* Instructions and forms you need to give someone legal control of your finances.

- *How to Probate an Estate* (California only). A simple explanation of how to read a will, handle probate paperwork, collect life insurance and other benefits, pay bills and taxes and distribute property left through trusts.

- *IRAs, 401(k)s & Other Retirement Plans: Taking Your Money Out.* How to tap into IRAs, 401(k)s and other retirement plans and get the most from them.

- *A Legal Guide for Lesbian and Gay Couples*. A complete guide to understanding the specialized interpretations and laws that affect gay couples, this book includes a chapter on estate planning concerns.

- *The Living Together Kit*. A legal and estate planning guide geared to the needs of unmarried heterosexual couples.

- *Make Your Own Living Trust.* A guide to living trusts—a popular device used to avoid probate. Includes forms and instructions for setting up two kinds of trusts: a basic probate avoidance trust and a more complex AB trust to save on estate taxes.
- *9 Ways to Avoid Estate Taxes.* Explains the nine major ways people can avoid, or reduce, federal estate taxes.
- *Nolo's Will Book.* All the forms and instructions needed to create a legally valid will, with examples of clauses to use to tailor your will to your own needs.
- *Plan Your Estate.* A thorough explanation of estate planning goals and techniques—including information on trusts. Shows how to prepare a complete estate plan without the expensive services of a lawyer. Considerable detail on federal estate taxes and strategies to avoid them.
- *The Quick and Legal Will Book.* Allows you to create a will on your own, without delay, fuss—and without hiring a lawyer.

Software

- *Nolo's Personal RecordKeeper.* Provides structure for a complete inventory of all your important legal, financial, personal and family records.
- *Living TrustMaker.* Helps you create your own living trust to avoid probate.
- *WillMaker.* Assists users in making several important legal documents: a will, healthcare directives, durable power of attorney for finances and final arrangements.

A. The Basic Need: A Will

Despite their own best interests, and often despite their own best intentions, many people do not have a will—the legal document that directs how to parcel out a person's property after death. And others may have a will drawn up so long ago that it no longer accurately reflects the will-maker's wishes, assets or family circumstances.

If you die without leaving a will, you are said to die "intestate." Your property will then be distributed to your spouse, children or other relatives if you have no spouse or children, according to the statutory formula or "intestate succession laws" in your state.

Even if you opt to transfer your property to others using other techniques such as a probate-avoiding living trust, preparing a simple will is an essential first step to planning any estate. In a will, not only do you spell out who you want to get your property, you can also name a personal representative (executor) to round up and distribute that property and to wind up your business and financial affairs after your death. A will also provides an opportunity for you to name a personal guardian for your own minor children and to name someone to manage property for any minor or young adult child to whom you leave property—until they reach an age you believe they will be capable of managing it alone.

Note that a "living will," discussed in Chapter 8, is something completely different from the kind of will discussed here. Living wills let you express your wishes about medical treatment in case you become ill or incapacitated; they are not devices to transfer property after death.

B. Avoiding Probate

Probate is the legal process by which a person's property, called an "estate," is distributed after death. It involves filing a will, if there is one, with the local probate court; identifying and appraising all the person's property; and paying debts and estate taxes and distributing what's left of the property according to the instructions in the will or according to state law if there is no will—all with the approval of the court. Except for small estates in the wide range of $5,000 to $60,000, depending on the state, and, in some states, for property left from one spouse to the other, all property left by a will must go through probate.

Fees for lawyers, appraisers, accountants and the probate court, which often total 5% to 7% or more of the value of the deceased person's estate, reduce the property that ultimately goes to the beneficiaries.

Another problem is that probate usually takes nine to eighteen months to complete and requires time and effort by the executor or administrator who is responsible for collecting and then distributing the estate property. Because of the cost and inconvenience of probate, many people arrange for distribution of their property through legal devices that avoid probate. Several of these methods—joint tenancy, pay-on death accounts, life insurance, living trusts and retirement accounts—are discussed briefly below, with special attention to their implications for estate planning for older people.

1. Joint Tenancy

Joint tenancy is one of the most popular probate avoidance devices. For many, joint tenancy is an easy way to prepare to handle simple finances—maintaining bank accounts, paying household bills—when the elder is no longer capable of doing so. Somewhat different rules apply to joint tenancy property in different states and it goes by different names—"tenancy by the entirety" for joint tenant married couples in some states; other states require the use of the term "right of survivorship."

In a joint tenancy, two or more people own the same property equally. Joint tenancy carries with it the "right of survivorship." This means that when one joint tenant dies, his or her share of the joint tenancy property automatically passes to, and becomes owned by, the surviving joint tenants. They need not go through probate or other legal gyrations to get full ownership of the property.

Joint tenancy is particularly useful as a management device for relatively small assets such as joint bank accounts. And, for older people, it may offer some convenience. If an elder becomes ill and is unable to get to the bank or becomes unable to manage his or her affairs, for example, a joint tenant on the account can take care of the finances without having to go through complicated bank or court procedures.

In most states, joint tenancy is easy to set up and can be done without an attorney, and without cost, by filling out a simple form available at the bank, stock brokerage or other financial institution that holds the assets.

Because each joint tenant has equal access to funds, there is always the danger that one joint tenant will misuse them, especially if large amounts are involved. Accordingly, joint tenancy is advisable only when there is complete trust between joint tenants. Older people, many of whom are vulnerable to those eager to defraud them of their assets, should be on the look-out for those who attempt to entrap them into suddenly changing ownership of their property.

In some states, you can protect against the risk of misuse by opening a joint tenancy bank account that requires the signatures of both joint tenants before withdrawals can be made. The problem with this arrangement, though, is that much of the convenience of joint tenancy is lost. If both signatures are required, joint tenancy funds would not be easily available if the elder becomes incapacitated.

Because property held in joint tenancy passes automatically at death, it also can be a useful probate avoidance tool for couples and other long-term co-owners of property who want the survivors to get their share. However, transferring solely owned property into joint tenancy is not usually the best method to avoid probate.

First, the IRS often considers a transfer of solely owned property into joint tenancy to be a taxable gift. If the new joint tenant did not pay full market value for his or her share, the transaction is legally considered to be a gift. With real estate, in particular, the gift is considered to be legally made when the new joint tenant is listed on the deed and it is recorded with the county land records office. If the value of the gift exceeds $10,000, a federal gift tax return must be filed by the giver of the gift. The exception is that money placed in a joint bank account is not a gift until the other person removes some of the money.

When the giver dies, the full market value of the real estate, as of the giver's death, is included in the giver's taxable estate, even though a half-interest was already given away during the giver's life. The giver's estate receives a tax credit for the gift tax previously assessed.

Using a living trust to achieve this goal avoids possible problems with a gift tax return because there is no transfer until the original owner dies. (See Section B5.) However, transferring solely owned property into joint tenancy can be useful as a last minute probate avoidance device, when death is imminent, if no living trust has been prepared and there is not sufficient time to prepare one.

Also, placing property in joint tenancy does not protect an asset in the face of Medicaid eligibility rules. As discussed in Chapter 6, these rules force an elder to spend most of his or her assets before Medicaid will begin to pay anything for a nursing facility or long-term care. But if assets are large enough, it makes good sense to take steps other than putting them in joint tenancy to protect them from these Medicaid rules. (See Chapter 7 for a detailed discussion of how to protect assets.)

2. Pay-on-Death Accounts, Stocks and Bonds

Most banks and savings institutions let depositors name someone to receive the contents of an account free of probate at the depositor's death. The depositor keeps sole control of the account during his or her lifetime, but whatever is in the account then passes to the beneficiary upon the depositor's death. Often called pay-on-death accounts or informal trusts, they provide a simple way of passing on money without having it go through probate.

However, this arrangement is not helpful if the depositor becomes incompetent, since no one else has access to that account during the depositor's lifetime. A durable power of attorney naming another person to handle financial matters can, however, be used to give him or her legal access to the account in the event the depositor becomes incompetent. (See the discussion of durable powers of attorney in Chapter 8.)

Some types of federal securities—and many stocks, bonds and mutual funds—also permit the owner to make a pay-on-death designation of a beneficiary. Whether or not you can make a pay-on-death designation depends on the state in which you live, the type of stock or security and the broker who handles the account. If you want a pay-on-death designation for your stocks, for example, but your broker cannot or will not set it up for you, consider hiring a different broker who will find a way to get the job done.

3. Life Insurance

Life insurance is another way to transfer money with no need for probate. This is because you name the beneficiary of the policy in the policy itself, and not in your will. The only time the property will be subject to probate is if you name your estate as the beneficiary on the policy. That set-up is made occasionally if the estate will need immediate cash to pay debts and taxes, but it is fairly uncommon. (See Section C1 for a discussion of making a gift of life insurance while you are alive to save on estate taxes.)

4. Retirement Accounts

Retirement accounts such as IRAs, 401(k) plans and Keogh accounts were not originally intended to be probate avoidance devices, but they can easily be used that way. All you do is name a beneficiary to receive the funds still in your pension plan or retirement account at your death, and the funds will not pass through probate.

After you reach age 70, however, federal law requires you to withdraw a minimum amount every year or face a monetary penalty. The amount you must withdraw is recomputed every year, based on your life expectancy.

5. Living Trusts

A trust is a legal entity, created by a document. It has the legal capacity to own property. Money or other property owned by a trust may be spent only according to the terms of the document that established the trust.

Trust assets are managed by someone called the "trustee," appointed by the person who sets up the trust, who is called the "trustor" or "settlor." Legally, a trustee can be any competent adult. For most living trusts, however, the trustor appoints himself or herself as trustee. This allows the elder who sets up the trust to keep full control over the trust property—and avoid probate, too.

The trust document also names a successor trustee to take over if the elder becomes incapacitated or dies. The trustee or successor trustee must administer the trust according to the elder's written trust instructions, which can be changed or revoked at any time, as long as the elder is competent. Upon the elder's death, the successor trustee distributes the assets according to the elder's trust instructions. This process functions very much like a will but without probate.

Example. *Tony wants to leave his valuable painting collection to his son and his home to his daughter, but wants to have and enjoy all the paintings and to continue to live in his home during his own lifetime. He also does not want the value of his extensive collection and real property—which are worth nearly $1 million combined—to be included in his probate estate when he dies. Tony takes care of all these concerns by establishing a living trust for the paintings, naming himself trustee while he lives, with his son the beneficiary of the paintings and his daughter of the house. He names his trusted friend Mavis as successor trustee. When Tony dies, Mavis will transfer the painting collection and house to his children outside of probate.*

There are a number of advantages to a revocable living trust. While alive, the trustor retains complete control over the assets. And instructions to a trustee can be as specific or as general as the elder wants. Because the trust can be controlled by the elder—either as trustee, by changing trust instructions, or by adding or subtracting trust assets—there is no risk of misuse of the funds as there is with a joint tenancy, which actually makes the eventual inheritor a co-owner of the property. Trust assets are also protected in the case of incapacity, because the successor trustee is normally empowered to handle them according to instructions. At death, assets are distributed to inheritors free of probate.

In many situations, simple living trusts can be set up without the use of an attorney and administered by a friend or relative as trustee. More complicated living trusts, however, may require an attorney to establish and to make later changes, and a bank or attorney to act as trustee.

> ### REVOCABLE LIVING TRUSTS AND MEDICAID
>
> If a living trust is revocable, its assets are not exempt from Medicaid eligibility limits. However, it is possible to create a revocable living trust with specific instructions to the trustee to transfer assets in a way that will get the most Medicaid eligibility and require the least in payment to a nursing facility. Those instructions must be very carefully written to take advantage of the asset protection methods which may be available to you as described in Chapter 7.

C. Saving on Estate Taxes

If you, or you and your spouse have a combined estate worth a relatively small amount, you will not likely be affected by federal estate tax concerns. However, if your estate, or the combined estate of you and your spouse exceeds a certain amount, you may face a hefty estate tax liability. Marginal tax rates begin at 37% for the first non-exempt dollar and go up fairly rapidly from there.

Fortunately, given fairly recent changes to the law, estate tax liability is less of a concern than it once was. For deaths in 1998, the tax credit is equal to the amount of estate tax assessed on an estate worth $625,000. So someone who dies in 1998 can leave up to $625,000 of property free of federal estate tax. The tax credit will increase for the next several years—meaning that fewer and fewer estates will be liable for estate taxes. The exact amounts are listed below.

THE PERSONAL ESTATE TAX EXEMPTION

YEAR	AMOUNT THAT CAN BE LEFT TAX-FREE
1998	$625,000
1999	$650,000
2000–2001	$675,000
2002–2003	$700,000
2004	$850,000
2005	$950,000
2006 and after	$1,000,000

Fortunately, in addition to the basic exemption, there are several other important estate tax exemptions. The most significant exemption is for property left to a surviving spouse. Quite simply, all property left to a surviving spouse who is a U.S. citizen is exempt from federal estate taxes. But caution: For larger estates, the fact that no federal estate tax is assessed may lead to a substantial tax liability when the second spouse dies. (See Section 1 below for a discussion of how a marital trust can help deal with this.)

The other main exemptions from estate tax are:

- the expenses of a last illness;
- burial costs;
- probate fees and expenses;
- certain debts, including a credit for state death taxes and death taxes imposed by foreign countries on property the deceased person owned there; and
- all tax-deductible charitable gifts made in a will.

1. Marital Trusts

A type of trust called a marital life estate trust, which can be established under a will or as part of a living trust, is one of the simplest ways to provide for management of funds with the added advantage, in some circumstances, of saving money on estate taxes. With a marital life estate trust, the elder completely controls the use of the assets during his or her lifetime. Upon the elder's death, the assets in the trust are administered by a trustee named by the elder under the terms specified in the will.

A marital trust works like this: Income from trust property, and in some cases the property itself, is left for the use of the surviving spouse during the other's lifetime, but the survivor never actually becomes the legal owner of the property. Since legal ownership bypasses the surviving spouse, the obligation of that spouse's estate to pay estate tax on the money received from the first spouse to die is also bypassed.

A marital trust is especially advisable for an elderly couple who has combined assets over the normal threshold at which federal estate taxes must be paid. If they each leave all their property to each other, with the surviving spouse then leaving the entire estate to other inheritors (such as their children), the total estate taxes will be based on all non-exempt property over the tax-credited amount for the year. The way a marital trust can save on taxes is that it allows each member of the couple to use his or her entire estate tax exemption. It prevents the surviving spouse from ending up with all the property belonging to both spouses and may save the survivor's estate a hefty estate tax liability.

2. Gifts

An excellent way to reduce your estate tax liability is to reduce the size of your estate by giving property to the same people you would ultimately like to leave it to anyway. Because gifts are taxed at the same rate as money left in an estate, savings can be realized by making a number of small gifts—as many as you want to and can afford to give—that are less than the annual $10,000 gift tax exemption. Here are some of the basic rules:

- As a gift, you can pay for another person's school tuition or medical bills in any amount, without incurring any gift tax liability. This payment can be on behalf of any person, but it must go directly to the school for tuition, or directly to the medical provider for medical bills. You cannot directly reimburse an individual for the amount of such a gift; if you do, it will be subject to gift tax.

- You can make a gift of any amount to your spouse without gift tax liability. To make sure that the money will not be counted as part of your estate, check with a tax attorney or accountant about the marital property rules in your state.

- You can make a gift of any amount to tax-exempt charities. Make certain that you have a written conformation—an acknowledgment with the organization's federal tax identification number on it—when you make any such gift.

GIFTS OF INSURANCE

The proceeds of life insurance are included in your estate for federal estate tax purposes if you own the policy. If you think your estate will be liable for federal estate taxes at your death, you can reduce the tax bill by transferring ownership of the policy before your death. This is a particularly good strategy because gift tax liability is imposed on the cash value of the policy at the time it is given, which is likely to be substantially less than its pay-off value at death. Once you have transferred ownership of the policy, the proceeds will not be counted as part of your taxable estate.

To satisfy the Internal Revenue Service that you have authentically transferred ownership of a life insurance policy, you must verify that you have given up total interest in the policy; you cannot keep the right to name beneficiaries, cancel coverage, borrow against the policy or make payments on it.

One final twist: You must transfer ownership of the policy—usually by completing a few simple forms you can get from your insurance company—at least three years before your death, or the IRS will count it as part of your taxable estate.

In making $10,000 annual gifts, it is a particularly good idea to give property that is likely to go up in value in the future. Otherwise, the increase in value would add to the net worth of the elder's estate if it goes over the untaxed limit.

3. State Death Taxes

About half the states impose death taxes on:

- all real estate owned in the state, no matter where the deceased person lived, and
- all other property of residents of the state, no matter where the property is located.

Home is where the tax is. Your taxability will be assessed in the state deemed your "legal residence." To establish a legal residence in a particular state, register all vehicles there, keep bank accounts there and vote in that state.

STATES WITHOUT DEATH TAXES

The states listed here take a cut of any federal tax paid. They do not impose an additional tax.

Alabama	Hawaii	Oregon
Alaska	Illinois	Texas
Arizona	Maine	Utah
Arkansas	Minnesota	Vermont
California	Missouri	Virginia
Colorado	Nevada	Washington
District of Columbia	New Mexico	West Virginia
Florida	North Dakota	Wyoming
Georgia		

If you live in a state that does not impose death taxes and you do not own real property in a state that imposes them, they need be of no concern to you. But if you spend different parts of the year in more than one state, it will allow your inheritors to take your personal property free of state inheritance tax if you establish your permanent legal residence in a state that does not have the taxes.

Example. *Harry and Margot, an elderly married couple, spend their winters in Florida and summers in New York. Florida has no death taxes. New York imposes comparatively stiff estate taxes—with rates ranging from 2% for $50,000 or less to 21% for $10,100,000 or more. It probably makes good sense for Harry and Margot to make Florida their legal residence. To do this, they should register to vote in Florida and conduct as many business transactions there as possible—for example, using Florida banks and registering vehicles in Florida. It might also make sense for them to sell any real property located in New York and simply rent when they are in that state.*

D. Managing Property

Ongoing trusts can be used to provide for the management and control of property when a person doesn't want to turn that property over to the beneficiary outright. Some beneficiaries, such as minors or people who have been declared legally incompetent, are not permitted to control substantial amounts of property on their own. Or the beneficiary may be seriously disabled, a spendthrift or have drug or alcohol abuse problems—all situations that may make it feasible for another person to be appointed property manager through a trust with the power to dole out money to the spendthrift on a periodic basis.

Property management trusts are a good option for an older person who wishes to pass property to someone who fits into one of these categories. With managerial trusts, it is particularly important to select a responsible trustee, someone who is attuned to the beneficiaries' needs. This is because the trustee will have an ongoing relationship with the beneficiaries and will also have important decisions to make, such as how to invest trust money and whether to expend part of the trust principal to meet special needs of the beneficiary.

SPECIAL CONCERNS FOR SUBSEQUENT MARRIAGES

People who marry more than once may face problems reconciling their desires for their present spouse and family with their wishes to be sure to pass property to the children from their prior marriages. Individual situations vary drastically, and you must carefully evaluate your desires to tailor your legal set-up to your situation.

Example. *Gertrude, a widow, has three grown children, owns a house and has other substantial assets. In her 70s, Gertrude marries Ted, also in his 70s. Ted has very little property and has two children from a prior marriage who Gertrude feels are both spoiled and ungrateful. As she plans her estate, Gertrude realizes that she wants to allow Ted to remain in the house if she dies before he does, but does not want him to be able to lease the property to his pushy kids. Understandably, Gertrude's own children share her concerns.*

Gertrude decides to give some of her property outright to her children. She also decides to create a trust for the house and to leave enough money in that trust to pay for the mortgage and upkeep on the house. The trust will specify that Ted has the right to live in the house for his lifetime, with the house to go to Gertrude's kids at Ted's death.

COMPARISON OF ASSET PROTECTION DEVICES

	Will	Joint Tenancy	Pay-on death Account	Trust under Will	Living Trust	Power of Attorney
Elder retains control of assets	yes	shared	yes	yes	yes	yes
Avoids probate	no	yes	yes	yes	yes	N/A
Can be set up easily without an attorney	yes	yes	yes	no	yes	yes
Automatic protection of assets under Medicaid	no	no	no	maybe[1]	no	no
Permits transfer of assets to protect re Medicaid	yes	yes	no	yes[2]	yes	yes[2]
Possible tax benefits	yes	yes	no	yes	yes	no
Protection if elder becomes incompetent	no	no	no	no	yes	yes
Can be revoked by elder	yes	no	yes	yes or no[3]	yes	yes[4]

[1]If the trust is revocable.

[2]If the written document specifically permits the trustee or attorney-in-fact to make such transfers.

[3]Can be created as a revocable or irrevocable trust.

[4]If it is a "springing" power of attorney. ■

Long-Term Care Insurance

Over the past decade, people have become increasingly aware of how easily long-term care can wipe out a lifetime's savings—and insurance companies have been quick to capitalize on that fear. Long-term care insurance, also called nursing home insurance, has been widely advertised as protection against the costs of long-term care, particularly against the costs of nursing facilities. But for the most part, this kind of insurance is expensive and provides only limited benefits—with many restrictions and conditions—that in many cases cover only a small percentage, or nothing at all, of total long-term care costs.

A. Risks and Benefits

Insurance companies market long-term care (LTC) insurance by suggesting to people that they are likely to wind up spending years in a nursing facility—a prospect that would wipe out their life's savings and perhaps leave them without a roof over their heads. The actual odds of such a long nursing facility stay, however, are considerably lower than the insurance industry would like you to imagine. And with the protection afforded by Medicaid laws, there is virtually no risk of being thrown out of a nursing facility and into the street. (See Chapters 4 and 6.)

When the true odds of a long nursing facility stay are considered along with the high cost of LTC insurance and the other uses to which the money for premiums could be put, you may find that for you—as for the 95% of the population over age 65 that has not invested in it—LTC insurance is not a good bet.

Nonetheless, there are a few people—for example, those who have assets of over $200,000 beyond the value of their homes—for whom LTC insurance may be a sound idea. This is particularly true if it is viewed as a safety net rather than a financial investment—and if

it includes coverage for assisted living facilities. (See Chapter 3.)
Those who do buy LTC insurance make the purchase at a median age
of 65. Before that age, most people's financial and health future is too
unpredictable for this insurance to make sense; by their 80s, the
premiums are usually unaffordable.

The odds of a long nursing facility stay. The true figures about how
much time a person is likely to spend in a nursing facility present a
rather different picture than the one painted in dark and somber
tones by the insurance industry.

- Two-thirds of all men, and one-third of all women, age 65 and
  older, will never spend a day in a custodial care nursing facility.
- Of people age 65 and over, only about 15% of men and 30% of
  women spend more than a year in a nursing facility.
- For stays of more than three years, the numbers are considerably
  lower: only 10% to 15% of all nursing facility residents stay that
  long.
- Of people who do enter a nursing facility, the average stay is about
  18 to 20 months.

The performance of long-term care insurance. The relatively long odds
against needing three or more years of nursing facility care have
meant that the insurance industry has not had to pay out on its
policies to nearly the extent that they suggested when they sold them.
And when the policies' conditions, exclusions and benefit limits are
figured in, the performance of these policies—at least in the decade
up to the mid-1990s, for which statistics are available—has been
quite poor.

- About 50% of all policies lapsed before any benefits were paid;
  people were unable or unwilling to continue paying their premiums.
- Of people who bought the insurance and later entered a nursing
  facility, about half never collected a dollar from their LTC policies.

- No benefits were ever paid to the many who bought nursing facility coverage but received home care or entered a residential facility not covered by the insurance, instead.
- When benefits were paid, they were far below the actual cost of care.
- For many of the longest-term residents, benefits were used up before the nursing facility stay ended.

In all of these situations, the LTC insurance failed to live up to its promise of keeping people from having to use up their savings, or to rely on Medicaid, to pay for long-term care. In other words, it was a lousy investment.

Improvements in LTC insurance. In response to pressure from consumer groups, to some embarrassing media exposure and to increased competition from other insurers joining the market, new LTC policies improved somewhat in the second half of the 1990s. Those improvements included clearer terms and conditions, so that people were better informed about what they might and might not get for their money.

Also, many policies extended coverage to include some types of assisted living residences, not just nursing facilities. (See Chapter 3.) Many policies now permit a pool of benefit funds to be used for either home care or residential care, rather than only one or the other. The requirements to qualify for benefits also have been loosened somewhat. And policies now routinely permit the policy holder to "step down" to lower levels of coverage, for a lower premium, if continuing to pay for the higher benefits becomes too financially burdensome.

If you are considering long-term care insurance, be a very careful consumer before you buy. Comparison shop among several policies and check each policy carefully for the exclusions and limitations discussed in this chapter. If you find one or two policies that you seriously consider, remind yourself that you may never need long-term care at all, and that if you do, it may not be for a long enough period to collect much in the way of insurance benefits. Before making a final decision, check with an accountant or financial adviser about whether some other types of secure long-term investments—with which you have more control and take less risk—might build up a fund of similar size as these particular insurance policies, but which you would use to pay for long-term care only if you need it.

The only way you can determine whether long-term care insurance is a good value for you is to gauge how much you are likely to pay in premiums before requiring home care or entering a facility—based on your age and general health. Remember, if you are buying a policy when you are in your 60s, you are likely to be paying premiums for 20 years or more before you might need long-term care. Measure that amount against the benefits you are likely to collect and the costs of care that would remain unpaid by the policy. Since what you are protecting against is the cost of substantial long-term care, make your calculations based on estimates of the cost in your geographic area. Estimate the costs in 10, 20 and 30 years from now of a three-year and six-year period of home care and a one-year, two-year and three-year residence in a nursing facility. Then consider, too, that you might never need extensive long-term care, and that in that case the policy will wind up paying you little or no benefits.

The 5% of income rule

Consumer and financial experts generally agree that long-term care insurance is a bad investment—in addition to the other reasons discussed in this chapter—unless you can pay the monthly premium with no more than 5% of your income. When calculating this 5% figure for future years, bear in mind that your premiums are likely to rise, while at some point your income will probably drop. (See Sections E1 and E2.)

In general, if in addition to your home, you expect to have substantial assets and income—over $100,000 in assets and over $30,000 per year in income—when you reach your 80s, then a long-term care policy with high benefits and compounded inflation protection might be a reasonable investment while you are in your 50s to early 70s if you can find and qualify for a good one based on the provisions described below.

In addition to the information insurance brokers and agents have, you may want to check the latest analysis of long-term care policies done by *Consumer Reports*, a consumer information magazine. The magazine regularly does comprehensive studies of specific long-term care policies and may be a valuable reference for you. *Consumer Reports* can be found at any local library.

However, even if you do expect to have sizable assets, a financial adviser may show you more profitable ways of investing the same money you would put into insurance premiums. And those investments plus permissible transfers of assets under Medicaid rules may combine to provide better protection and liquidity for your money than a long-term care insurance policy. In any event, do not base your decision solely on advice from an insurance agent or broker who is trying to sell you a long-term care policy.

LONG-TERM CARE INSURANCE NOW TAX DEDUCTIBLE

Health insurance premiums have long been tax deductible as medical expenses. And health insurance benefits were not considered income. Long-term care insurance premiums and benefits, however, were not given the same treatment because they were not technically for care defined as medical. As of January 1, 1997, however, a certain amount of long-term care insurance premiums may be deductible as medical expenses—to the extent they, like other medical deductions, exceed 7.5% of your gross adjusted income. And benefits under a long-term care insurance policy will not be considered as income.

For its premiums to be deductible and its benefits not to be treated as income, a policy must meet federal guidelines that identify it as Qualified Long Term Care Insurance (QLTCI).

If you enrolled in your policy before 1997, it is automatically considered a QLTCI for tax purposes. After January 1, 1997, a new QLTCI policy must identify itself as "intended to meet the federal requirements."

The maximum amount per year of QLTCI policy premiums that can be deducted as a medical expense depends on your age:

Age	Amount Deductible
40 years and under	$200
40 to 49	$375
50 to 59	$750
60 to 69	$2,000
70 and over	$2,500

These tax law amounts change regularly, so check the instructions on your federal tax return for the current figures.

SEVERAL STATE POLICIES NOW HELP PROTECT ASSETS

California, Connecticut, Indiana and New York Medicaid programs have special arrangements by which Medicaid and private insurance companies cooperate to offer long-term care policies protecting a greater measure of assets than are normally allowed when Medicaid covers long-term care. The asset-protection aspects of these special long-term care policies are described in Chapter 7, Section B8.

Beware that the mere fact that these policies might protect some assets is not enough automatically to make them a good investment. All the other requirements for a good long-term care policy, as explained in this chapter, also apply to these asset-protection policies.

B. Warnings About Insurance Practices

It can be a mind-boggling task to shop for any kind of insurance, but those searching for long-term care insurance should be armed with the following special warnings.

Beware of pretty numbers. Don't be blinded by the first numbers you are shown by an insurance advertisement, agent or broker. Very often, a company will flash at you what seem like low premiums and high benefits, as if premiums and benefits for all people for all coverage were the same, and as if premiums and benefits were the only matters that count. If you pay the premiums and never see the benefits, you'll know too late that there are other important questions, discussed in this chapter, to ask before buying a policy.

Beware of brochures and agents. Insurance brochures and advertisements are often misleading and are always incomplete. Brochures and ads are intended to get you interested in insurance policies and to convince you how great they are—not to explain their pitfalls and problems or even to explain accurately how they work. And brochures that are not detailed enough do not bind an insurance company to anything in particular, so you cannot rely on their glossy general promises.

Insurance agents, too, are in the business of selling policies—not of warning you why you should not buy one. Although most agents are conscientious about not selling a policy they know is not right for a customer, some will say almost anything to make a sale. Other agents may not intentionally mislead you, but sell you a bad policy simply because they do not know better. Long-term care insurance is relatively new and policies change rapidly, so many agents simply do not have much experience with or understanding of particular policies and coverages.

In general, an insurance agent—as opposed to an insurance broker—represents only one company or group of companies. He or she may know that company's policies fairly well but can offer you no other company's insurance with which you can compare premiums and coverage. If you have received information from one company's agent, even if the agent has shown you that company's "different" policies, be sure to investigate several other companies' policies as well. Also, do not rely on what an agent tells you about how a policy works. An agent does represent the company, but if you are going to rely on something the agent tells you, insist that you see the promise in writing on the policy itself or from the agent or other company representative in an official company correspondence addressed to you.

An insurance broker, as opposed to an agent, works independently and can offer policies from a number of different companies. A broker can probably show you a somewhat wider selection of long-term care policies than could an agent who works for only one company. A broker may not know very well how the different policies operate, however. And nothing a broker says is considered binding against the insurance company, so if the broker contends that a policy operates in a certain way, again, be sure you see it in writing on the policy or in official correspondence from the company to you.

Beware of mail-order and limited-time-only policies. You have probably seen these advertising catch-phrases before; they often come unsolicited in the mail: Limited Offer! Once-in-a-Lifetime! When this offer expires, you'll never get the same chance again! One Month Only!

These one-time-only offers are usually misleading nonsense. The best advice may simply be to avoid buying any policy touted in an advertisement that uses an exclamation point. If it is a reputable insurance company with a legitimate policy to offer, the same or similar terms will be available to you at any time—except for premium increases because of a change in your age. No matter what the advertising says, don't be rushed into buying anything.

Check the company's reliability rating. No insurance policy is any good if the company who issued it has gone bankrupt by the time you try to collect your benefits. An independent insurance industry guide called *Best's Insurance Reports* rates individual insurance companies as to general reliability and financial health. Consider buying a policy only from an insurance company with a *Best's* rating of A+ or A. *Best's* is often available at your local library, but if you have trouble finding a recent copy, the insurance agent or broker you deal with concerning the long-term care policy, or any other insurance broker, should be able to get you a written statement of the company's *Best's* rating.

Remember, however, that even a high *Best's* rating is no guarantee of a foolproof policy. If you buy now, you may not need to collect benefits under the policy for 15, 20 or 25 years. And there is no way anyone can predict the financial health of a particular insurance company over that period. This uncertainty is yet another reason to consider other forms of long-term investment instead of long-term care insurance.

Examine the policy. When you seriously consider a particular long-term care insurance policy, don't be content to just look at a summary of it. Examine the entire policy—and not in the insurance agent or broker's office. Take it home so that you can study it carefully and have family, friends or a financial adviser check it with you.

After reading the policy carefully, ask the agent or broker any questions you have about any aspect of the policy—premiums, coverage, exclusions, benefits—and request responses in writing, signed, either directly from the company or by the agent stating that he or she is responding on behalf of the company. These responses cannot come from an independent broker, but must be from someone who officially represents the insurance company. Ask for some evidence that the person who is giving you the explanation is authorized to speak on behalf of the company. If you do choose to purchase a policy based on such an extra written explanation, make sure that the written explanation is attached to and made an official part of your policy.

C. Extent of Coverage

The long-term care you or a loved one may need at some point could take one of several forms—and over time, even more than one form. Initially, long-term care might mean regular but not daily help at home with some of the routine activities of daily living (ADLs). Or, it could mean 24-hour monitoring and care in a nursing facility. Or it might encompass any level of at-home or residential care in between.

Some LTC policies cover nursing facility care, but not home care. Others cover home care only. And some comprehensive policies cover not only those two types of care, but also assisted living in some facilities. When you consider LTC insurance, look for policies covering the broadest types of care that might be useful to you. And be sure to determine what benefits will be provided, and for how long, at each separate level of care.

1. Custodial Care Nursing Facilities

Unless you are interested in a policy for home care only (see Section C3, below), your main concern will be coverage for a long stay in a nursing facility. A policy should state clearly that coverage is for custodial care.

The other main consideration is the way the policy defines the facilities in which the policyholder is eligible to receive coverage. Eligibility restricted to facilities licensed by the state as custodial care nursing facilities presents no problem. But avoid any policy that requires a facility to be certified by Medicare. Medicare covers only skilled nursing care, and many nursing facilities that provide custodial care do not provide skilled care and so would not have Medicare certification. Beware, too, of any requirement regarding the size of the facility. A few policies will not cover care in facilities with less than a certain number of beds, usually 20 or 30. But there is no reason a small facility cannot provide excellent care, and such a limited-bed facility in your area might be exactly the type of place that would best suit your needs.

2. Assisted Living Facilities

One of the most important developments in long-term care in recent years has been the rise of assisted living residences as an alternative to nursing facilities. They provide part-time personal assistance and monitoring for people who need some help with the activities of daily life but who do not need the intensive care and monitoring of a nursing facility. (See Chapter 3, Section B.) And now LTC insurance, which before had covered only nursing facilities and home care, is catching up with this change.

One of the first things to investigate about any policy is whether it covers assisted living residences, and the terms under which it does. How the policy refers to these non-nursing facility residences is not important; they go by several names. (See Chapter 3, Section B.) And a policy may fairly require some state licensing or certification.

What matters are the specific conditions under which a policy holder may qualify for coverage. (The events that trigger coverage are explained in Section D, below.) The policy should use the same triggers for assisted living as it does for a nursing facility. Your decision about whether to move to an assisted living facility or a more restrictive, institutional and expensive nursing facility should be based on your personal needs and preferences, not on whether an insurance policy will cover you.

RESIDENTIAL COVERAGE WITHOUT HOME CARE

Some people may want to consider a policy that provides residential nursing facility coverage, but not home care. If you are unmarried, do not have younger family members close by who can be counted on to help you if you stay at home, and you live in an area with few home or community care services available, home care might not be a realistic alternative for you and there seems little point in paying extra for its coverage.

However, if the cost of adding home care is not too great, the extra coverage might be worth the extra expense. By the time you need long-term care—10, 15, 20 years from now—home and community care may have become a much more viable alternative for you than it would be now.

---

3. Home and Community Care

Many insurance companies provide coverage for certain types of long-term home care and care provided at non-resident community care facilities, either in the same policy as residential facility coverage or as a separate home-care-only policy. Because home and community care is becoming available in more places, and with broader and more innovative services, home and community care coverage in a long-term care policy makes good sense for most people.

Home and community care coverage only. Some people may want to consider home and community care coverage only, without any residential facility coverage.

You may want to consider home care coverage only without the more expensive residential nursing facility coverage, if:

- you are considerably older or more physically limited than your spouse, and she or he is capable of caring for you at home if the need should arise; your spouse, though should have residential care coverage;
- you have other supportive family who live nearby and would help with care;
- or, you have adult children who are willing and able to take you into their homes to care for you if the need should arise and you prefer that arrangement to living in a residential facility; and
- you live in an area with many home and community care services available; or
- you do not have large assets (over $100,000) other than your home which you seek to protect from nursing home costs. (See Chapter 7.)

Remember, though, that you are insuring for a need which may not arise for ten, fifteen or twenty years—and it is difficult to predict what your situation will be at that time. If you choose to purchase home and community care coverage only, be sure also to pay attention to the protection of your assets from nursing home costs under Medicaid rules. (See Chapter 7.)

Broadest possible coverage. As discussed in Chapter 2, home care covers a wide variety of services, from fairly intensive nursing and physical or speech therapy, to help with activities of daily living (ADLs) such as bathing, eating, moving about, to homemaker services such as housecleaning, shopping and laundry. If you seek long-term home care insurance, try to get the widest variety of coverage possible. There are a number of conditions and restrictions of which you should be aware.

- Some policies cover only skilled nursing care and physical therapy in the home, but not custodial care. Such coverage is far too limited and should be rejected.

- Most home care policies cover custodial care provided by trained home health aides who work for a licensed home care agency—not the much more expensive care provided by nurses or medical therapists.

- A few policies also provide limited coverage of some homemaker services if those services are provided by an agency home health aide in addition to other personal assistance duties.

- Some policies cover care provided not only in the home, but also in licensed community care facilities such as adult day care centers.

- Very few policies cover any services if provided by independent aides rather than through a licensed home care agency.

Disability Home Care Plans

A few insurance companies have begun to offer what are called disability plans for home care benefits. You will probably have to shop extensively to find a policy that has this kind of payout and that also meets your other criteria.

Usual disability policies require that the insured receive a particular type of care, or care only from specified categories of caregiver.

Disability coverage requires merely that the insured make a claim that he or she is "disabled" as defined by the policy—usually meaning that the insured cannot perform without assistance a certain number of activities of daily living (ADLs) as listed in the policy.

The insurance company then confirms the disability by checking the insured's medical records and receiving a certification of disability from the insured's doctor—and sometimes having one of their own doctors examine the insured. Once the disability level is confirmed, the insurer pays out the policy benefits directly to the insured who can use it any way he or she wants.

D. Coverage Conditions and Exclusions

The main risk in purchasing a long-term care insurance policy is the great likelihood that you will pay premiums for many years, but will never require care for a long enough period to collect substantial insurance benefits. But policies also present other barriers to collecting benefits. The many terms, conditions and exclusions in long-term care policies sometimes eliminate coverage for people who need it most. You must consider these conditions—particularly the most common ones discussed below—very carefully when shopping for a policy.

1. Prior Hospital or Skilled Nursing Facility Stay

One of the insurance industry's cruelest tricks during the early days of long-term care coverage was to hide in the small print of a policy the condition that the policy would pay benefits only if the long-term care began within a short period—usually 7 to 30 days—after the

insured's three-day stay in a hospital or skilled nursing facility (SNF).
Some custodial care does immediately follow a hospital or SNF stay.
Most long-term custodial care, however, is for chronic illness, frailty,
Alzheimer's disease or physical or mental impairment and does not
follow an acute medical episode which resulted in a three-day or
longer hospital or SNF stay.

Most states have now banned this prerequisite of a three-day
hospital or SNF stay. However, in about a quarter of the states, such
provisions are still legal and it is up to you as a consumer to spot such
a provision in a policy which is offered to you. Specifically ask the
insurance agent or broker whether such a provision exists in any
policy shown you. Do not buy any policy with a requirement of a
prior hospital or skilled nursing facility stay.

BEWARE OF PERMANENT EXCLUSIONS

A few policies permanently exclude coverage if you enter a nursing facility or begin receiving home or community care as a result of a specific illness or medical condition. The effect of such an exclusion is that you would receive no benefits, no matter how long you received care.

The conditions excluded are usually mental illness, HIV-related illness, nervous disorders, alcohol or chemical dependency, certain heart diseases, certain forms of cancer and diabetes. If your need for long-term care arises from any of these or other conditions permanently excluded from the policy you have purchased, it will not pay any benefits toward the cost of that care.

If you already know that you have suffered from one of the excluded conditions listed in a particular policy, it is obvious that this policy is no good for you. But, you should also avoid any policy that has a long list of exclusions even though at this point in your life you have never had any of the listed illnesses or conditions. You may not need the policy coverage for many years—and in those intervening years, you may develop one of the listed illnesses or conditions which will lead to a need for long-term care.

2. Pre-Existing Condition Exclusion

Like other health-related insurance policies, some long-term care policies exclude coverage for care required by an illness or condition diagnosed or treated within a certain time—usually six months to two years—before the start of the policy.

The exclusion may work in any of several ways. Some policies exclude coverage for a certain time after you begin receiving long-term care. During that exclusion period, the insurance company would pay no benefits for your care. If this period is relatively short—three to six months—it may not be too severe a restriction on coverage. If the exclusion is for a longer period—for one year, for example—you would be greatly increasing the probability that you will never receive any benefits under the policy. Look for a policy with no exclusion at all. If you must accept an exclusion, look for a combination of the shortest pre-care period and the shortest exclusion period.

3. Qualifying for Benefits: Necessity of Care

Beginning to receive a type of care described in a long-term care insurance policy does not necessarily begin coverage. Instead, most long-term care policies have some sort of standard the insured must meet to qualify for benefits. This standard usually requires a doctor to certify that you have a medically related need for the care. And how that need is defined in the policy, as well as which doctor decides if it has been met, can be crucial to whether you receive the benefits for which you have paid.

Medically necessary care. One of the standards that long-term care policies use to determine whether an insured has qualified for benefits is that the care the insured is receiving is medically necessary due to illness or injury. This standard can present several problems.

■ How is illness defined? Simple frailty, or a combination of frailty and some disorientation or memory loss, is the most common cause of the need for long-term care, yet it may be very difficult to pinpoint a specific illness to which to attribute these conditions.

■ When does an illness or injury end? Even if a definable illness or injury has clearly caused the initial need for care, after a while, an insurance company may claim that the illness has ended or the injury healed and that care is now received for mere frailty or disorientation, neither of which is covered under the policy.

Be extremely wary of any policy that uses the "medically necessary due to illness or injury" standard. If the policy strongly interests you for other reasons, at least make sure of two things.

First, be sure that the definition of "illness or injury" is as broad as possible, including loss of mental faculties or mental disorientation as well as specific mention of Alzheimer's disease.

Second, be sure that your personal physician, rather than a doctor appointed by the insurance company, makes the initial determination of the medical necessity of care—although almost all policies have a provision that allows a second opinion by a company doctor to challenge your own physician's opinion.

Performing activities of daily living. A much better standard—and an increasingly more common one—than "medically necessary due to illness or injury" is the "inability to perform without assistance" some of the activities of daily living or ADLs. Each insurance policy has its own list of five to seven different ADLs including eating, bathing, dressing, using the toilet, getting in and out of bed or chair, taking medication and walking around. Each policy also sets its own number of ADLs with which the policyholder must need assistance before benefits begin.

When considering a policy that uses ADLs as a standard, look for the following requirements and conditions.

■ In some policies, coverage goes into effect if assistance is needed with only two ADLs; in other policies three. It is obviously better for you if only two are required.

■ It is particularly important that only two ADLs be required if the policy list of ADLs includes a total of only five; a requirement of three ADLs is easier to meet if there are a total of seven ADLs listed.

■ Bathing is almost always one of the first ADLs with which people need help; bathing should always be included in the list of qualifying ADLs.

■ Check whether there is a different number of ADLs required to qualify for coverage of separate levels of care—for example, only two ADLs for home care, but three for assisted living or nursing facility care. Try to get the fewest number of ADLs for each level of care.

■ A good policy should be clear that the "inability to perform without assistance" includes the ability to perform sometimes, but not without supervision.

Mental competence tests. Good policies also offer a test of the insured's mental competence—often referred to as cognitive abilities—as an alternative to the physical ADLs standard. This alternative test qualifies for benefits those insured who are physically able to perform ADLs but who are mentally incapable of regularly performing them. This is a crucial additional policy term because it is mental condition—without any severe accompanying physical disability—that gives rise to the need for long-term care for many people.

E. Premiums and Terms of Renewal

The cost of premiums and terms of renewal are two prime characteristics to search out and understand in any long-term care policy.

1. Initial Premium Cost

The cost of initial premiums varies with your age and overall health as well as with the quality, amounts and length of coverage. If you are in the 50 to 59 age group, you may be able to get a long-term policy with small benefits over a limited period for less than $1,000 per year. If you are over 70 and want broad coverage and sizable benefits payable for several years, a new policy may cost $7,000 per year.

If your purpose in purchasing long-term care insurance is to protect your income and assets from the high cost of long-term care, then it only makes sense to buy coverage if it will be high enough and last long enough to make a serious dent in those costs. If your benefits cover only a small percentage of your long-term care costs, those costs will eat up all your savings anyway and you will have spent money on years of premiums for nothing. So, as a rule, small benefits (under $100 day for residence facility care) and a limited coverage period (less than two years) is of questionable value, particularly as to nursing facility costs. Anything less than these benefits is probably a poor investment.

In addition to your age and the size of the benefits, however, less obvious things like the number of conditions and exclusions, the levels of care, benefit flexibility and inflation protection (see Section F3), as well as waiver of premiums, terms of renewal or premium hikes and premature death refunds, will all affect the amount of premiums on any specific policy.

2. Terms of Renewal or Premium Hikes

All long-term care policies are now guaranteed renewable, which means that an insurance company cannot simply drop your policy if it decides a particular line of coverage is not profitable. Problems still exist, however, with the terms under which you are permitted to continue coverage year after year.

Insist on level premiums. Insurance companies do not guarantee that your premiums will not go up over time. All they will promise is that premiums will be raised only across the board—and that yours will remain the same as that for others with the exact same policy who purchase it at the same age and same time. However, there is some additional protection in policies that guarantee level premiums. Level premiums will not automatically rise as you get older, although the insurance company is still free to raise its rates across the board for all policy holders.

Avoid attained-age premiums. One of the ways insurance companies entice customers to a particular policy is to offer very low initial premiums while hiding in the fine print the fact that the premiums will rise automatically when the insured attains certain age levels— usually 70, 75, 80 and 85. With such attained-age premium rises, after ten or 15 years, the premiums could be so high that you can no longer afford them and you will be forced to drop your coverage— wasting all the money you've paid in premiums—when you are most likely to need the benefits.

STEP-DOWN PROVISIONS: GOOD EXTRA PROTECTION

One of the major problems with long-term care insurance is that policyholders may pay premiums for 20 or 30 years or more before they need benefits, and it may become very difficult for them to keep up financially. Premiums rise over time, incomes drop and other expenses may take over most of expendable income. Because of this slow deterioration of many older people's finances, over half of those holding LTC policies written in the mid-1980s to the early-1990s were forced to allow their coverage to lapse.

To help reduce the odds that this will happen to you, look for a policy that allows you to "step down" your coverage. A step-down means that the amount of the daily benefit the policy will pay, or the level of care it will cover, or the length of coverage, will be reduced from the amount for which you originally signed up. In exchange, the insurance company lowers your premium by a certain percentage. This may make it possible to keep the policy in effect—although for a diminished benefit—if you have trouble meeting the more expensive original premium.

Policies with step-down provisions also sometimes permit you to "step up" as well—to increase potential benefits in exchange for a higher premium. However, many policies require a step-up to be underwritten—meaning that you must still be in good health to move to higher benefits. A step-up provision may be of particular interest to someone who is young and doesn't want to take on high premiums until he or she is sure that the financial future will be rosy enough to pay for them, but who wants to leave open the option to pay for higher benefit protection.

3. Waiver of Premiums

A very important, but sometimes overlooked, provision in long-term care policies is known as waiver of premiums. This means that after a period during which you are collecting certain benefits under the policy, you stop paying premiums. This is an important provision because otherwise, most of the benefits you receive may just go back to the insurance company in the form of premiums.

Waiver of premiums more often applies to residential care benefits only, and not to home care. A few policies offer premium waivers as soon as benefits begin, although most require that you continue paying premiums for the first 30 to 90 days you receive benefits. As with most other policy terms, the better the waiver of premiums provision, the higher your initial premiums will be.

SPECIAL RULES FOR ALZHEIMER'S PATIENTS

Most states now have regulations that require all long-term care policies to provide benefits to those insured who require care due to medically diagnosed Alzheimer's disease. The problem is that there is no clear medical test to determine when someone has Alzheimer's disease rather than some other form of mental disorientation.

If you have a policy that requires a medically definable illness, but does not specifically cover mental disorientation or consider the performance of ADLs, you may have a difficult time proving the existence of Alzheimer's as the cause of the need for care. On the other hand, if you have a policy that begins benefits if the insured cannot perform a certain number of ADLs, Alzheimer's alone may not qualify you if you are still physically able to perform those activities, as are many Alzheimer's patients.

The best solution to this Alzheimer's coverage problem is to have the broadest possible policy definition of need for care, to have a mental competence test as an alternative qualifying standard, and to have a policy that permits you and your own doctor to decide whether you need care.

F. Benefit Amounts

Unlike most health insurance, almost all long-term care policies pay a fixed amount for each level of care regardless of, and usually well below, the actual cost. Benefits vary from $25 to $250 per day—with a given policy's benefits for nursing facility care usually twice as much as it pays for home care and benefits for assisted living somewhere in between. Of course, the amount of benefits depends on how high a premium is charged. But the actual amount you wind up receiving can also depend on your careful purchase of a policy that has benefit flexibility, a limited "elimination" or waiting period and inflation protection.

1. Flexible Benefit Pay-Out

Long-term care policies have a limit on the total dollar value of benefits they will pay, determined by the amount of daily benefits multiplied by the length of coverage you purchase—for example, $100/day for three years of residence facility care or $50/day for six years of home care = $109,500. If you have coverage of both nursing facility care and home care or of nursing facility, assisted living and home care, it is a great advantage to have a policy that will pay its maximum benefits in any combination, sometimes called a pool of coverage. You should be able to use your benefits on one level of care, then switch to another level and use whatever total amount of benefits remains unpaid. Do not get a policy that forces you to choose between one level of care or another, or that will not pay for a different level of care if you later need it.

Take, for example, a policy with a maximum benefit of $109,500—$50/day for six years of home care, $100/day for three years of nursing facility care. You would want flexible benefit terms in that policy that permit you to use three years of home care benefits amounting to $54,750 ($50/day for 1,095 days) and leave the remaining amount (another $54,750) for use in a residential facility ($100/day for 547 days).

It is also preferable to have a policy that is flexible regarding the time period by which it measures home care benefit amounts—that is, by the week, month or year, not merely by the day. This may be important if the daily cost of your home care exceeds your daily benefit amount, but you don't get the care every day. For example, if you receive $100 per day worth of home care three days a week, a policy that only pays $75 per day would leave you with $25 per day unpaid for each of the three days of care. On the other hand, if your policy was flexible and paid either by the day or week—$75 per day or $525 per week (7 days x $75/day = $525)—then the policy would cover the full amount of your $300 per week home care costs.

2. Elimination or Waiting Period

Almost all long-term care policies have a waiting period, called an elimination or deductible period, immediately following a claim for benefits during which no benefits are paid. During that period— ranging from ten days to one year following the beginning of care— you are responsible for paying all your long-term care costs. Generally, the longer the elimination period, the lower your premiums. An elimination period of six months to one year may reduce your premiums by as much as one-third.

In many instances, the need for care—either at home or in a nursing facility—is relatively short and there is a relatively long elimination period during which you might not receive any benefits at all. However, the real purpose of a long-term care policy is not to have insurance cover the costs of a short period of care, but to prevent the asset-devouring, impoverishing costs of a long period of expensive care. Therefore, a longer elimination period—90 days to six months—probably makes good sense if it results in substantial premium savings. This is particularly true if you are buying the policy when you are in your 50s or 60s and therefore will probably be paying the premiums for a long time.

3. Inflation Protection

A benefit of $100 per day for residential care probably seems reasonable given today's average nursing facility costs of $40,000 to $50,000 per year. But you are not buying a policy to protect yourself against today's long-term care costs. You are buying a policy to protect against the costs of care 10, 20, or 30 more years from now when you are far more likely to need its coverage. Since the cost of medical care widely outpaces the overall cost of living, custodial care in a nursing facility 10 years from now could easily cost $300 per day; 20 years from now who knows how high the cost will be? If your benefits then are still only $100 daily, the uncovered costs would eat up your personal assets at lightening speed and your years of paying long-term care insurance premiums would be wasted.

The only way to protect yourself from such skyrocketing costs is to make sure your long-term care policy has good inflation protection built into it. And the key here is to get good inflation protection, because it comes in several different forms.

■ *Added coverage purchase*. This type of provision permits you every few years to purchase added coverage with higher benefits. The problem with this is that the added coverage will also come with new premiums— based on your increased age plus any other rate increases—that you may not be able to afford. You may find yourself with benefits too low to be useful but without the means to buy added coverage, with the result that you wind up dropping the insurance just as you reach an age when you might need decent coverage.

■ *Simple automatic increase*. Many policies offer benefits which increase by a fixed percentage—usually 5%—or by each year's national cost-of-living increase, but they always use the original benefit amount as the base which the percentage increase is measured. These policies are better than the added coverage purchase option, discussed above, because your benefits go up automatically without requiring higher premiums.

- *Compounded automatic increase.* These policies automatically increase benefit amounts each year by a set percentage or by the cost-of-living increase, and they compound the increases each year rather than always using the original benefit amount as a base figure. Over 10 to 20 years, this compounding might make a tremendous difference in your benefits. Of course, because automatic compounded inflation protection is so much better for the insured, the premiums for such coverage are usually considerably higher from the beginning.

- *Time limited protection.* Most policies put a time limit on the yearly inflation benefit increase. The limit is usually 10 to 25 years from the date the policy begins, or when the insured reaches a certain age, usually 80 or 85. If you buy the policy when you are in your 50s or 60s, it is important to get the longest possible period of inflation protection.

Good inflation protection may raise the initial cost of a policy by 25% to 50%. But without good inflation protection, the lower premiums may be a total waste of money.

G. Refund Provisions

There are several reasons why you might end your long-term care policy before full, or any, benefits are paid—a change in your financial picture, a sharp increase in premiums, a change in health or death. What becomes of all those years of premiums you have paid but never collected on?

As with life insurance, a few long-term care policies permit the refund of some of your premiums if your coverage ends before full benefits have been paid. These are not offered in many policies—

most often in group policies—and do not provide any great financial protection. Therefore, they should not be major considerations in deciding on a policy. But, if you are trying to decide between two policies which are close in most important categories, the existence of one or another of these refund provisions might tip the balance.

1. Non-Forfeiture Provisions

These provisions require that if you drop your coverage before you have collected benefits under the policy, some percentage of your equity in the policy—that is, the total amount of premiums you have paid—will be returned to you. The amount is usually quite small and there is most often a requirement that the policy must have remained in effect for a certain period of time—10, 15, 20 years. A non-forfeiture provision may be most attractive to someone young, whose future is uncertain but likely long.

2. Reduced Paid-Up Provisions

These provide that after you have paid premiums for a specified number of years (usually 20 or 25), you can drop your coverage—that is, stop paying premiums—but still collect reduced benefit amounts when you otherwise qualify for benefits.

3. Death Refunds

These terms provide that if an insured dies before a certain age (usually 65 or 70), then a small percentage of the premiums paid (less any benefits paid) will be returned to the insured's estate.

4. Survivorship Provisions

These provisions give some protection to a surviving spouse when both spouses have purchased LTC policies. With a survivorship clause, if one insured spouse dies, the surviving spouse may stop paying premiums after a set number of years, but the insurance will remain in effect. This can be very important if the death of one spouse drastically reduces the amount of the couple's income. ■

Appendix

Resource Directory

Aging, State Offices

These are the central offices in each state, run by the state government, which provide general information and referrals to all the specific agencies within the state which provide services for elders.

ALABAMA

Commission on Aging
770 Washington Street, Suite 470
Montgomery, AL 36130
334-242-5743

ALASKA

Senior Services Division
Department of Administration
Box 110200
Juneau, AK 99811-0209
907-465-3250

ARIZONA

Aging & Adult Administration
Department of Economic Security
1789 West Jefferson, Suite 950A
Phoenix, AZ 85007
602-542-4446

ARKANSAS

Division of Aging, Adult Services
Department of Social Rehabilitative Services
P.O. Box 1437
7th and Main Streets
Little Rock, AR 72201
501-682-2441

CALIFORNIA

Department on Aging
1600 K Street
Sacramento, CA 95814
916-322-5290

COLORADO

Aging and Adult Services Division
110 16th Street
Denver, CO 80202
303-620-4147

CONNECTICUT

Department on Aging
25 Sigourney Street
Hartford, CT 06106
860-424-5277

DELAWARE

Division on Aging
Department of Health and Social Services
1901 North Dupont Highway
New Castle, DE 19720
302-577-4791

DISTRICT OF COLUMBIA

Office on Aging
441 Fourth Street, NW
Washington, DC 20001
202-724-5622

FLORIDA

Department of Elder Affairs
4040 Esplanade Way
Tallahassee, FL 32399-7000
904-414-2000

GEORGIA

Office of Aging
Two Peachtree Street, NW
Atlanta, GA 30309
404-657-5258

HAWAII

Executive Office on Aging
250 South Hotel Street, Suite 107
Honolulu, HI 96813
808-586-0100

IDAHO

Office on Aging
3380 American Terrace, Suite 120
Boise, ID 83706
208-334-3833

ILLINOIS

Department on Aging
421 East Capitol Avenue, Suite 100
Springfield, IL 62701
217-785-2870

INDIANA

Department of Aging and Rehabilitative Services
402 West Washington Division
Indianapolis, IN 46204
317-232-7020

IOWA

Department of Elder Affairs
Clemens Building, 3d Floor
200 Tenth Street
Des Moines, IA 50309-3609
515-281-5187

KANSAS

Department on Aging
New England Building
503 South Kansas
Topeka, KS 66603-3404
785-296-4986

KENTUCKY

Division for Aging Services
Department of Human
  Resources
CHR Building, 6th Floor
275 East Main Street
Frankfort, KY 40621
502-564-6930

LOUISIANA

Office of Elder Affairs
P.O. Box 80374
Baton Rouge, LA 70898-0374
225-342-7100

MAINE

Bureau of Elder and Adult
  Services
Department of Human Services
State House, Station #11
35 Anthony Avenue
Augusta, ME 04333
207-624-5335

MARYLAND

Office on Aging
State Office Building
301 West Preston Street, Room
  1007
Baltimore, MD 21201
410-225-1100

MASSACHUSETTS

Executive Office of Elder Affairs
McCormack Building, 5th Floor
One Ashburton Place
Boston, MA 02108
617-727-7750

MICHIGAN

Office of Services to the Aging
611 West Ottowa Street, 3rd
  Floor
P.O. Box 30026
Lansing, MI 48909
517-373-8230

MINNESOTA

Board on Aging
444 Lafayette Road
St. Paul, MN 55155-3843
612-296-2770

MISSISSIPPI

Council on Aging
750 North State Street
Jackson, MS 39202
601-359-4925

MISSOURI

Division on Aging
Department of Social Services
P.O. Box 1337
615 Howerton Court
Jefferson City, MO 65102-
  1337
573-751-3082

MONTANA

Senior and Long Term Care
  Division
Department of Public Health
  and Human Services
P.O. Box 4210
111 Sanders, Room 211
Helena, MT 59604
406-444-7788

NEBRASKA

Department on Aging
301 Centennial Mall South
P.O. Box 95044
Lincoln, NE 68509
402-471-2307

NEVADA

Division on Aging
Department of Human
  Resources
340 North 11th Street, Suite
  203
Carson City, NV 89101
702-486-3545

NEW HAMPSHIRE

Division of Elderly and Adult
  Services
State Office Park South
115 Pleasant Street
Annex Building #1
Concord, NH 03301
603-271-4680

NEW JERSEY

Division of Senior Affairs
Department of Health and
  Senior Affairs
P.O. Box 807
Trenton, NJ 08625-0807
609-588-3141
800-792-8820

NEW MEXICO

State Agency on Aging
224 East Palace Avenue
La Villa Rivera Building
Santa Fe, NM 87501
505-827-7640

NEW YORK

Office for the Aging
Empire State Plaza
Agency Building #2
Albany, NY 12223
518-474-5731
800-342-9871

NORTH CAROLINA

Division on Aging
693 Palmer Drive
Raleigh, NC 27626
919-733-3983

NORTH DAKOTA

Aging Services
State Capitol Building
600 East Boulevard Avenue
Bismarck, ND 58505-0250
701-328-8910

OHIO

Department on Aging
50 West Broad Street, 8th Floor
Columbus, OH 43215-5928
614-466-5500

OKLAHOMA

Aging Services
Department of Human Services
P.O. Box 25352
312 N.E. 28th Street
Oklahoma City, OK 73125
405-521-2327

OREGON

Senior Services Division
500 Summer Street, NE
Salem, OR 97310
503-945-5811

PENNSYLVANIA

Department on Aging
555 Walnut Street
Harrisburg, PA 17101-1919
717-783-1550

PUERTO RICO

Governor's Office of Elderly
Affairs
Call Box 50063
Old San Juan Station, PR
00902
787-721-5710

RHODE ISLAND

Department of Elderly Affairs
160 Pine Street
Providence, RI 02903
401-277-2858

SOUTH CAROLINA

Governor's Division on Aging
P.O. Box 8206
Columbia, SC 29201
803-253-6177

SOUTH DAKOTA

Office of Adult Services
700 Governors Drive
Pierre, SD 57501-2291
605-773-3656

TENNESSEE

Commission on Aging
Andrew Jackson Building
500 Deaderick Street
Nashville, TN 37243-0860
615-741-2056

TEXAS

Department on Aging
4900 North Lamar, 4th Floor
Austin, TX 78751
512-424-6840

UTAH

Division of Aging and Adult
Services
Human Services Department
120 North 200 West, Room
401
Salt Lake City, UT 84145
801-538-3910

VERMONT

Aging and Disabilities Department
Human Services Agency
103 South Main Street
Waterbury, VT 05676
802-241-2400

VIRGINIA

Department for the Aging
1600 Forest Avenue, Suite 102
Richmond, VA 23219-2327
804-662-9333

WASHINGTON

Aging and Adult Services
Administration
Department of Social and
Health Services
P.O. Box 45050
Olympia, WA 98504-5050
360-586-8753

WEST VIRGINIA

Office on Aging
Holly Grove, State Capitol
1900 Kanawha Boulevard East
Charleston, WV 25305-0160
304-558-3317

WISCONSIN

Aging Bureau
Community Services Division
P.O. Box 7851
Madison, WI 53707
608-266-2536

WYOMING

Commission on Aging
117 Hathaway Building
Cheyenne, WY 82002
307-777-7986

Caregiver Support Groups

Children of Aging Parents
1609 Woodbourne Road, #302A
Levittown, PA 19057
800-227-7294

A nonprofit organization that provides support and information to
the families and friends of the dependent elderly. It maintains a
directory of self-help support groups for family caregivers, publishes a
number of pamphlets for caregivers and puts out a newsletter that
provides information on programs for the elderly and their families.
Enclose $1 and a self-addressed, stamped envelope with any request
for information.

National Family Caregivers Association
10605 Concord Street, Suite 501
Kensington, MD 20895-2504
800-896-3650

A membership group that publishes a newsletter for family caregivers,
provides referrals and conducts a caregiver-to-caregiver support
network. Also publishes a caregiver resources guide, available
through the organization.

Home Care, Community Programs and Senior Residences

The following organizations provide information, and some give referrals to specific providers and facilities, regarding home care agencies, community senior services and non-nursing home senior residences. They can also put you in touch with state and local organizations, which can in turn provide you with even more detailed information and referrals.

Following this list of national organizations is a list of state associations that provide information on home care.

National Organizations

Aging Network Services
Topaz House
4400 East-West Highway, kSuite 907
Bethesda, MD 20814
301-667-4329

Alliance for Children and Families
(formerly Family Service America)
1701 K Street NW, Suite 200
Washington, DC 20036-1503
202-223-3447
Offers senior referrals as well as other family services.

Alzheimer's Association
919 North Michigan Avenue, Suite 1000
Chicago, IL 60611-1676
800-272-3900
312-335-8700
National association that makes referrals to local support groups.

American Federation of Home Health Agencies
1320 Fenwick Lane, Suite 100
Silver Springs, MD 20910
301-588-1454

American Hospital Association
Division of Ambulatory Care
840 North Lake Shore Drive
Chicago, IL 60611
312-280-6216

The Eldercare Locator
800-677-1116
Open Monday through Friday, 9 a.m. to 8 p.m. (EST), referring
people to eldercare services in communities across the country.

Health Hotlines
Public Information Office
National Library of Medicine
Bethesda, MD 20894
Offers a directory of local hotlines that provide free help for people
coping with a variety of health problems associated with aging.

Health Information Center
P.O. Box 1133
Washington, DC 20013
800-336-4797

Joint Commission for Accreditation of Health Care Organizations
One Renaissance Boulevard
Oakbrook Terrace, IL 60181
630-792-5000
FAX: 630-916-5644

National Association for Home Care
228 Seventh Street, SE
Washington, DC 20003
202-547-7424

National Association of
Professional Geriatric Care Managers
1604 North Country Club Road
Tucson, AZ 85716
520-881-8008

National Council on the Aging
409 3rd Street
Washington, DC 20024
202-479-1200
800-424-9046

National Hispanic Council on Aging
2713 Ontario Road, NW
Washington, DC 20009
202-265-1288
Provides information on topics related to Hispanics and aging, and
provides particular assistance for Spanish-speaking seniors.

National Parkinson Foundation
1501 NW 9th Avenue
Miami, FL 33136
305-547-6666
800-327-4545

Visiting Nurse Association Hospice Care
1260 Andes Boulevard
St. Louis, MO 63132
314-993-1280

State Associations

ALABAMA

Alabama Association of Home
  Health Agencies
P.O. Box 40
Montgomery, AL 36101
334-832-1400

ALASKA

Alaska Home Care Association
c/o Valley Home Care
950 East Bogard, Suite 133
Wasilla, AK 99654-7172
907-352-2845

ARIZONA

Arizona Association for Home
  Care
2334 McClintock Drive
Tempe, AZ 85282
602-967-2624

ARKANSAS

Home Care Association of
  Arkansas
501 Woodlane, Suite 100
Little Rock, AR 72201
501-376-2273

CALIFORNIA

California Association for
  Health Services at Home
723 S Street
Sacramento, CA 95816-6209
916-443-8055

COLORADO

Colorado Association of Home
  Health Agencies
7853 East Arapahoe Road, Suite
  2100
Englewood, CO 80112
303-694-4728

CONNECTICUT

Connecticut Association for
  Home Care
110 Barnes Road
P.O. Box 90
Wallingford, CT 06492-0090
203-265-9931

DELAWARE

Delaware Association of Home
  Care and Community Care
Veale Road Professional Center
309 Veale Road
Wilmington, DE 19810
302-529-3000

DISTRICT OF COLUMBIA

Capitol Home Health Association
5151 Wisconsin Avenue, NW,
  Suite 400
Washington, DC 20016-4124
202-686-8728

FLORIDA

Associated Home Health
  Industries of Florida
820 East Park Avenue, Building
  H
Tallahassee, FL 32301-2600
904-222-8967

GEORGIA

Georgia Association of Home
Health Agencies
320 Interstate North Parkway,
Suite 490
Atlanta, GA 30339-2203
770-984-9704

HAWAII

Hawaii Association for Home
Care
1471 Pule Place
Honolulu, HI 96816
808-735-2970

IDAHO

Idaho Association of Home
Health Agencies
P.O. Box 6508
Boise, ID 83707
208-887-0916

ILLINOIS

Illinois Home Care Council
222 West Ontario, Suite 430
Chicago, IL 60210
312-335-9922

INDIANA

Indiana Association of Home
Care
8888 Keystone Crossing, Suite
1000
Indianapolis, IN 46240
317-844-6630

IOWA

Iowa Association for Home
Care
1520 High Street, Suite 203-B
Des Moines, IA 50309
515-282-3965

KANSAS

Kansas Home Care Association
1000 Monterey Way, Suite E2
Lawrence, KS 66049
785-841-8611

KENTUCKY

Kentucky Home Health
Association
154 Patchen Drive, Suite 90
Lexington, KY 40517
606-268-2574

LOUISIANA

Home Care Association of
Louisiana
233-A East Main Street
New Iberia, LA 70562
318-560-9610

MAINE

Home Care Alliance of Maine
20 Middle Street
Augusta, ME 04841
207-623-0345

MARYLAND

Maryland National Capital
Homecare Association
1738 Elton Road, Suite 312
Silver Spring, MD 20903
301-408-4005

MASSACHUSETTS

Home & Health Care Association of Massachusetts
20 Park Plaza, Suite 620
Boston, MA 02116
617-482-8830

MICHIGAN

Michigan Home Health
Association
2140 University Park Drive,
Suite 220
Okemos, MI 48864
517-349-8089

MINNESOTA

Minnesota Home Care
Association
1711 West County Road B,
Suite 209N
St. Paul, MN 55113-4036
612-635-0607

MISSISSIPPI

Mississippi Association for
Home Care
661 Highway 51 North, Suite 1B
Ridgeland, MS 39157
601-853-7533

MISSOURI

Missouri Alliance for Home
Care
2420 Hyde Park Road, Suite A
Jefferson City, MO 65109
314-634-7772

MONTANA

Montana Association of Home
Health Agencies
1905 River Road
Missoula, MT 59801
406-883-8442

NEBRASKA

Nebraska Association of Home
and Community Health
Agencies
14506 South Circle
Omaha, NE 68137
Phone: n/a

NEVADA

Home Health Care Association
of Nevada
P.O. Box 12190
Reno, NV 89510-2190
702-323-6003

NEW HAMPSHIRE

Home Health Care Association
of New Hampshire
8 Green Street
Concord, NH 03301
603-225-5597

NEW JERSEY

Home Health Services and
   Staffing Association of New
   Jersey
510 Ocean Avenue, Suite 31
West End, NJ 07740
732-870-6277

NEW MEXICO

New Mexico Association for
   Home Care
3200 Carlisle Boulevard, NE,
   Suite 115
Albuquerque, NM 87110
505-889-4556

NEW YORK

Home Care Association of New
   York State
21 Elk Street
Albany, NY 12207
518-426-8764

NORTH CAROLINA

North Carolina Association for
   Home & Hospice Care
226 West Millbrook Road
Raleigh, NC 27609
919-848-3450

NORTH DAKOTA

North Dakota Association of
   Home Health Services
P.O. Box 2175
Bismarck, ND 58502-2175
701-224-1815

OHIO

Ohio Council for Home Care
6230 Busch Boulevard, Suite 460
Columbus, OH 43229-1826
614-885-0434

OKLAHOMA

Oklahoma Association for
   Home Care
6303 North Portland, Suite 205
Oklahoma City, OK 73112-
   1411
405-943-6242

OREGON

Oregon Association for Home
   Care
147 Southeast 102nd Avenue
Portland, OR 97216
503-253-9237

PENNSYLVANIA

Pennsylvania Association of
   Home Health Agencies
20 Erford Road, Suite 115
Lemoyne, PA 17043
717-975-9448

PUERTO RICO

Puerto Rico Home Health
   Agencies and Hospices
   Association
P.O. Box 192152
San Juan, PR 00909-2152
809-774-8181

RHODE ISLAND

Rhode Island Partnership for
   Home Care
P.O. Box 603309
Providence, RI 02906
401-751-2487

SOUTH CAROLINA

South Carolina Home Care
   Association
P.O. Box 1763
Columbia, SC 29202
803-254-7355

SOUTH DAKOTA

South Dakota Association of
   Health Care Organizations
3708 Brooks Place
Sioux Falls, SD 57106
605-361-2281

TENNESSEE

Tennessee Association for
   Home Care
131 Donelson Pike
Nashville, TN 37214-2901
615-885-3399

TEXAS

Texas Association for Home
   Care
3737 Executive Center Drive,
   Suite 151
Austin, TX 78731
512-338-9293

UTAH

Utah Association of Home
   Health Agencies
6949 South High Tech Drive,
   Suite 150
Midvale, UT 84047
801-255-5888

VERMONT

Vermont Assembly of Home
   Health Agencies
10 Main Street
Montpelier, VT 05602
802-229-0579

VIRGINIA

Virginia Association for Home
   Care
5407 Patterson Avenue, Suite
   200B
Richmond, VA 23288
804-285-8636
800-755-8636

WASHINGTON

Home Care Association of
   Washington
23607 Highway 99, Suite 2C
P.O. Box C-2016
Edmonds, WA 98026
425-775-8120

WEST VIRGINIA

West Virginia Council of Home
  Health Agencies
Grand Central Station Drive,
  Suite 5011
Morgantown, WV 26505
304-292-5826

WISCONSIN

Wisconsin Homecare Organization
5610 Medical Circle, Suite 33
Madison, WI 53719
608-278-1115

WYOMING

Home Health Care Alliance of
  Wyoming
2600 East 18th Street
Cheyenne, WY 82001
307-778-5616

Insurance—Long-Term Care

The following are sources of information about what long-term care
insurance policies are available in your state.

Council for Affordable Health Insurance
112 South West Street
Alexandria, VA 22314
703-836-6200

American Association of Health Plans
1129 20th Street, NW, Suite 600
Washington, DC 20036
202-778-3200

Health Insurance Association of America
555 13th Street, NW, Suite 600 East
Washington, DC 20004
202-824-1600

State Departments of Insurance

Each state has a government agency that regulates the sale of insurance. There should be a listing for an insurance department under the

listings in the white pages of the telephone directory for Government Offices. It can provide you with a list of companies authorized to sell long-term insurance in your state.

State Offices on Aging

Like the Departments of Insurance, the Office on Aging in your state should have a current list of long-term care policies authorized for sale in your state. The Offices on Aging are listed earlier in this Resource Directory.

Legal Assistance

The following groups either provide, or give referrals for, protection of the legal rights of the elderly. Some provide information on government programs and legislation affecting the elderly. Others will refer you to lawyers in your area who specialize in legal matters affecting elders, such as reviewing the terms of a reverse mortgage, preparing powers of attorney and estate planning devices.

American Bar Association
Commission on Legal Problems for the Elderly
1800 M Street, NW
Washington, DC 20036
202-662-1000

Gray Panthers Project Fund
2025 Pennsylvania Avenue NW, #821
Washington, DC 20006
202-466-3132

Legal Counsel for the Elderly
American Association of Retired Persons
601 E Street, NW
Washington, DC 20049
202-434-2170

Legal Services for the Elderly Poor
130 West 42nd Street
New York, NY 10036
212-391-0120

National Academy of Elder Law Attorneys
1604 North Country Club Road
Tucson, AZ 85716
520-881-4005

National Caucus and Center on Black Aged
1424 K Street, NW
Washington, DC 20005-2410
202-637-8400

National Council of Senior Citizens
8403 Colesville Road, #1200
Silver Spring, MD 20910-3314
301-578-8800

National Senior Citizens Law Center
1101 14th Street, NW, #400
Washington, DC 20005
202-289-6976

Older Women's League
666 11th Street, NW, Suite 700
Washington, DC 20001
202-783-6689

60 Plus
1616 North Fort Meyer Drive
Arlington, VA 22209
703-807-2070

United Seniors Association, Inc.
3900 Jermantown Road, Suite 450
Fairfax, VA 22030
703-803-6747
800-887-2872

Licensing and Certification

Agencies on Nursing Care Standards

These are the agencies in each state that establish standards to be met by home health care agencies, nursing facilities and individual health care providers such as independent home health care workers. They can provide you with information regarding whether any particular health care provider or facility is licensed or certified by the state and what state standards must be met for that license or certification.

See also the list of Nursing Facility License and Certification Offices immediately following this one.

ALABAMA

Bureau of Licensing &
  Certification
Alabama Department of Public
  Health
434 Monroe Street
Montgomery, AL 36130-1701
334-240-3503

ALASKA

Health Facilities Licensing &
  Certification
Department of Health &
  Social Services
4730 Business Park Boulevard
Building H, Suite 18
Anchorage AK 99503
907-561-8081

ARIZONA

Health Care Institutions &
  Licensing
Department of Health Services
1647 East Morton Avenue,
  Suite 110
Phoenix, AZ 85020
602-255-1221

ARKANSAS

Medicare Certification
Arkansas Department of
  Health
5800 West 10th Street, Suite
  400
Little Rock, AR 72204
501-661-2201

CALIFORNIA

Licensing & Certification of
  Health Services
1800 3rd Street, Suite 210
Sacramento, CA 95814
916-445-2070

COLORADO

Health Facilities Regulation
  Division
Department of Public Health
  and Environment
4210 East 11th Avenue
Denver, CO 80220
303-331-6600

CONNECTICUT

Licensing & Certification
  Division of Hospital &
  Medical Care
Department of Health Services
150 Washington Street
Hartford, CT 06106
203-566-1073

DELAWARE

Health Facilities Licensing &
  Certification
Department of Health and
  Social Services
3300 Newport Gap Pike
Wilmington, DE 19808
302-995-6674

DISTRICT OF COLUMBIA

Service Facilities
Regulation Administration
Department of Consumer &
  Regulatory Affairs
614 H Street, NW, Suite 1003
Washington, DC 20001
202-727-7190

FLORIDA

Division of Health Quality
  Assurance
Office of Licensure and
  Certification
2727 Mahan Drive, Suite 214
Tallahassee, FL 32308-5407
904-487-2527

GEORGIA

Office of Regulatory Services
Health Care Section
Department of Human
  Resources
Two Peachtree Street, NW
Atlanta, GA 30303-3167
404-657-5550

HAWAII

Hospital & Medical Facilities
  Branch
Department of Health
P.O. Box 3378
Honolulu, HI 96801
808-586-4080

IDAHO

Facilities Standards Program
Department of Health and
  Welfare
P.O. Box 83720
Boise, ID 83720
208-334-6626

ILLINOIS

Division of Health Care
  Facilities and Programs
525 West Jefferson, 5th Floor
Springfield, IL 62761
217-782-7412

INDIANA

Division of Acute Care
Indiana State Department of
  Health
2 North Meridian Street
Indianapolis, IN 46204
317-233-7472

IOWA

Division of Health Facilities
Department of Inspections and
  Appeals
Lucas State Office Building, 3rd
  Floor
Des Moines, IA 50319
515-281-4115

KANSAS

Bureau of Adult & Child Care
Kansas Department of Health &
  Environment
Landon State Office Building,
  Suite 1001
900 SW Jackson Street
Topeka, KS 66612-1290
913-296-1280

KENTUCKY

Division for Licensure &
  Regulation
Cabinet for Human Resources
  Building
275 East Main Street
Frankfort, KY 40621
502-564-2800

LOUISIANA

Health Standards Section
Department of Health &
  Hospitals
P.O. Box 3767
Baton Rouge, LA 70821
504-342-0138

MAINE

Division of Licensure &
  Certification
Department of Human Services
State House Station 11
Augusta, ME 04333
207-624-5443

MARYLAND

Office of Licensure & Certifica-
  tion Programs
Department of Health & Mental
  Hygiene
4201 Patterson Avenue, 4th
  Floor
Baltimore, MD 21215
410-764-4980

MASSACHUSETTS

Division of Health Care Quality
Department of Public Health
80 Boylston Street, Suite 1100
Boston, MA 02116
617-727-5860

MICHIGAN

Bureau of Health Systems
Department of Public Health
3500 North Logan
P.O. Box 30195
Lansing, MI 48909
517-335-8505

MINNESOTA

Facility and Provide Compliance Division
Minnesota Department of
  Health
393 North Dunlap Street
St. Paul, MN 55164-0938
612-643-2130

MISSISSIPPI

Division of Health Facilities
  Licensure & Certification
Mississippi State Department of
  Health
P.O. Box 1700
Jackson, MS 39215
601-354-7300

MISSOURI

Bureau of Hospital Licensing
  and Certification
Missouri Department of Health
P.O. Box 570
Jefferson City, MO 65102
573-751-6302

MONTANA

Division of Quality Assurance
Department of Health and
  Human Services
Cogswell Building
1400 Broadway
Helena, MT 59620
406-444-2037

NEBRASKA

Department of Health
Division of Licensure &
  Standards
P.O. Box 94986
Lincoln, NE 68509-4986
402-471-2116

NEVADA

Bureau of Licensure and
  Certification
Nevada Health Division
1550 East College Parkway
Carson City, NV 89710
702-687-4475

NEW HAMPSHIRE

Administrative Division of
  Public Health Services
Bureau of Health Facilities
Six Hazen Drive
Concord, NH 03301
603-271-4592

NEW JERSEY

Licensure Certification &
  Standards
New Jersey Department of
  Health
CN360
Trenton, NJ 08625
609-292-5960

NEW MEXICO

Department of Health,
  Licensing and Certification
  Bureau
525 Camino de los Marquez,
  Suite 2
Santa Fe, NM 87501
505-827-4200

NEW YORK

Bureau of Hospital Services
Office of Health Systems
  Management
P.O. Box 7126
Albany, NY 12224
518-439-7286

NORTH CAROLINA

Department of Human
  Resources
Division of Facilities Services
701 Barbour Drive
P.O. Box 29530
Raleigh, NC 27626
919-733-7451

NORTH DAKOTA

Health Resources Section
600 East Boulevard Avenue
Bismark, ND 58505-0200
701-328-2352

OHIO

Bureau of Medical Services
Ohio Department of Health
246 North High Street
P.O. Box 118
Columbus, OH 43266-0588
614-466-7857

OKLAHOMA

State Commission of Health
Department of Health
1000 NE 10th Street
Oklahoma City, OK 73152
405-271-6576

OREGON

Health Care Licensure and
   Certification
Oregon Health Division
800 Northeast Oregon Street,
   Suite 640
Portland, OR 97232
503-731-4013

PENNSYLVANIA

Bureau of Quality Assurance
Pennsylvania Department of
   Health
Health & Welfare Building,
   Suite 532
Harrisburg, PA 17120
717-783-8980

PUERTO RICO

Health & Service Facilities
   Administration
Department of Health
P.O. Box 70184
San Juan PR 00936
809-766-1616

RHODE ISLAND

Division of Facilities Regulation
Rhode Island Department of
   Health
3 Capitol Hill, Room 306
Providence, RI 02908
401-277-2566

SOUTH CAROLINA

Division of Health, Licensure &
   Certification
Department of Health &
   Environmental Control
2600 Bull Street
Columbia, SC 29201
803-737-7202

SOUTH DAKOTA

Licensure & Certification
   Program
South Dakota Department of
   Health
615 East Fourth Street
Pierre, SD 57501
605-773-3356

TENNESSEE

Health Center Facilities
Department of Health
426 Fifth Avenue N.
Nashville, TN 37247-0508
615-741-7221

TEXAS

Health Facility Certification
Texas Department of Health
8407 Wall Street
Austin, TX 78754
512-834-6650

UTAH

Bureau of Health Facility
   Licensure
Department of Health
P.O. Box 142003
Salt Lake City, UT 84114-2003
801-538-6152

VERMONT

Department of Aging and
   Disability
103 South Main Street
Waterbury, VT 05671
802-241-2345

VIRGINIA

Office of Health Facilities
   Regulation
Department of Health
3600 Center, Suite 216
3600 West Broad Street
Richmond, VA 23230
804-367-2102

WASHINGTON

Washington Acute Care and
   Construction Review Services
Washington Department of
   Health
Target Plaza, Suite 500
2725 Harrison Avenue, NW
P.O. Box 47852
Olympia, WA 98504-7952
360-705-6780

WEST VIRGINIA

Health Facilities Licensure &
   Certification Division
West Virginia Department of
   Health
1900 Kanawha Boulevard East,
   Building 3
Charleston, WV 25305
304-558-0050

WISCONSIN

Bureau of Quality Compliance
Wisconsin Division of Health
One Wilson Street
P.O. Box 309
Madison, WI 53701
608-266-8481

WYOMING

Department of Health
Health Facilities Licensing
Metropolitan Bank Building,
   8th Floor
Cheyenne, WY 82002
307-777-7123

Nursing Facility License and Certification Offices

These offices are the government agencies in each state which inspect nursing facilities, issue state licenses and Medicare and Medicaid certifications. You can check the record of any nursing facility in the state through this office.

ALABAMA

Nursing Home Licensure Office
Division of Licensure and
   Certification
Alabama Department of Health
434 Monroe Street
Montgomery, AL 36130
334-240-3503

ALASKA

Nursing Home Licensure Office
Department of Health and
   Social Services
Health Facilities Certification
   and Licensing
4730 Business Park Boulevard,
   Building H, Suite 18
Anchorage, AK 99503
907-561-8081

ARIZONA

Department of Health Services
Office of Health Care Licensure
1647 East Morten
Phoenix, AZ 85020
602-255-1197

ARKANSAS

Arkansas Department of Health
Certification and Licensure
   Section
Office of Long-Term Care
Sixth and Louisiana Streets
P.O. Box 8059, Slot 400
Little Rock, AR 72203
501-682-8487

CALIFORNIA

Nursing Home Licensure Office
Licensure and Certification
   Division
Facilities Licensing Section
714 P Street, Room 823
Sacramento, CA 95814
916-657-1425

COLORADO

Nursing Home Licensure Office
Colorado Department of Public
   Health and Environment
   Department
Health Facilities Division
Evaluation and Licensure
   Section
4300 Cherry Creek Drive South
Denver, CO 80222
303-692-2800

CONNECTICUT

Nursing Home Licensure Office
Connecticut State Department
   of Health
Division of Hospital and
   Medical Care
150 Washington Street
Hartford, CT 06106
860-566-4800

DELAWARE

Office of Health Facility
   Licensing
and Certification
Nursing Home Division
Department of Health and
   Social Services
Three Mill Road, Suite 308
Wilmington, DE 19806
302-577-6666

DISTRICT OF COLUMBIA

Office of Licensing and
   Certification
Nursing Home Division
Department of Consumer and
   Regulatory Affairs
614 H Street, NW, Suite 903
Washington, DC 20001
202-727-7480

FLORIDA

Nursing Home Licensure Office
Licensure and Certification
   Branch
Division of Health
Department of Rehabilitation
   Services
2727 Mahan Drive
Tallahassee, FL 32308
904-487-2527

GEORGIA

Nursing Home Licensure Office
Standards and Licensure Unit
Office of Regulatory Services
Two Peachtree Street, NW,
    Suite 325
Atlanta, GA 30303
404-657-5700

HAWAII

Nursing Home Licensure Office
Hospital and Medical Facility
    Branch
Hawaii State Department of
    Health
P.O. Box 3378
Honolulu, HI 96801
808-586-4080

IDAHO

Nursing Home Licensure Office
Facilities Standards and
    Development
Idaho Department of Health
    and Welfare
P.O. Box 83720
Boise, ID 83720-0036
208-334-6626

ILLINOIS

Nursing Home Licensure Office
Illinois Department of Public
    Health
Health Facilities and Quality of
    Care
525 West Jefferson, Fourth
    Floor
Springfield, IL 62761
217-782-7412

INDIANA

Nursing Home Licensure Office
Division of Health Facilities
Indiana State Board of Health
2 North Meridian Street
Indianapolis, IN 46206-1964
317-233-7442

IOWA

Nursing Home Licensure Office
State Department of Inspections
    & Appeals
Division of Health Facilities
Lucas State Office Building, 3rd
    Floor
Des Moines, IA 50319
515-281-4115

KANSAS

Kansas Department of Health
    and Environment
Bureau of Adult and Child Care
Landon State Office Building
900 SW Jackson, Suite 1001
Topeka, KS 66612-1290
913-296-3362

KENTUCKY

Nursing Home Licensure Office
Division for Licensing and
    Regulation
CHR Building, Fourth Floor
    East
275 East Main Street
Frankfort, KY 40621-0001
502-564-2800

LOUISIANA

Nursing Home Licensure Office
Department of Health and
    Human Resources
Division of Licensure &
    Certification
P.O. Box 3767
Baton Rouge, LA 70821-3767
504-342-0138

MAINE

Nursing Home Licensure Office
Division of Licensure and
    Certification
35 Anthony Avenue
State House Station 11
Augusta, ME 04333
207-624-5443

MARYLAND

Office of Licensing and
    Certification Program
Department of Health and
    Mental Hygiene
4201 Patterson Avenue, 4th
    Floor
Baltimore, MD 21215
301-764-2750

MASSACHUSETTS

Nursing Home Licensure Office
Long-Term Care Facilities
    Program
Department of Public Health
150 Tremont Street
Boston, MA 02111
617-727-0201

MICHIGAN

Nursing Home Licensure Office
Bureau of Health Care Adminis-
    tration
Department of Public Health
525 West Ottowa
Lansing, MI 48909
517-241-2626

MINNESOTA

Nursing Home Licensure Office
Minnesota Department of
    Health
Survey and Compliance Section
393 North Dunlap Street
P.O. Box 64900
St. Paul, MN 55164-0900
612-643-2130

MISSISSIPPI

Nursing Home Licensure Office
Health Facilities Certification
    and Licensure
Mississippi State Board of
    Health
P.O. Box 1700
Jackson, MS 39215-1700
601-354-7300

MISSOURI

Missouri Department of Health
P.O. Box 570
Jefferson City, MO 65102
573-751-6336

MONTANA

Montana Department of Health
and Environmental Sciences
Bureau of Licensing and
Certification
Health Services Division
Cogswell Building
Helena, MT 59620
406-444-2037

NEBRASKA

Division of Licensure and
Standards
Nursing Home Division
Department of Health
301 Centennial Mall South
P.O. Box 95007
Lincoln, NE 68509
402-471-2946

NEVADA

Bureau of Licensure and
Certification
Nevada Health Division
1550 College Parkway
Capitol Complex, Suite 158
Carson City, NV 89710
702-687-4475

NEW HAMPSHIRE

Department of Health and
Human Services
Division of Public Health
Bureau of Health Facilities
Administration
Six Hazen Drive
Concord, NH 03301-6527
603-271-4592

NEW JERSEY

Nursing Home Licensure Office
New Jersey State Department of
Health
Licensing, Certification and
Standards
CN360
Trenton, NJ 08625
609-292-8773

NEW MEXICO

Nursing Home Licensure Office
Health Department
525 Camino de los Merquez,
Suite 2
Santa Fe, NM 87501
505-827-4200

NEW YORK

New York State Department of
Health
Bureau of Long Term Care
Services
Tower Building
Empire State Plaza, Room 1482
Albany, NY 12237
518-474-6462

NORTH CAROLINA

Nursing Home Licensure Office
Licensure and Certification
Section
Health Care Facilities Branch
701 Barbour Drive
Raleigh, NC 27603
919-733-1610

NORTH DAKOTA

Division of Health Facilities
State Department of Health
Nursing Home Division
State Capitol
600 East Boulevard Avenue
Bismarck, ND 58505
701-328-2352

OHIO

Nursing Home Licensure
Office
Medical Services
Licensing and Certification
Division
Ohio Department of Health
246 North High Street
Box 118
Columbus, OH 43266-0118
614-466-8739

OKLAHOMA

Nursing Home Licensure
Office
Licensure and Certification
Division
Oklahoma State Department of
Health
1000 NE Tenth
Oklahoma City, OK 73117
405-271-6576

OREGON

Oregon Health Division
Health Care Licensure and
Certification
P.O. Box 14950
Portland, OR 97214-0450
503-731-4013

PENNSYLVANIA

Nursing Home Licensure
Office
Commonwealth of Pennsylva-
nia
Division of Long-Term Care
Health and Welfare Building
Room 930
Harrisburg, PA 17120
717-787-8015

RHODE ISLAND

Nursing Home Licensure Office
Rhode Island Department of
    Health
Division of Facilities Regulation
3 Capitol Hill
Providence, RI 02908-5097
401-277-2566

SOUTH CAROLINA

Nursing Home Licensure Office
Division of Health Facilities and
    Services
Department of Health Licensing
2600 Bull Street
Columbia, SC 29201
803-737-7370

SOUTH DAKOTA

Department of Health
Division of Licensure and
    Certification
Anderson Building
445 East Capitol Street
Pierre, SD 57501-3182
605-773-3356

TENNESSEE

Department of Health and
    Environment
Board for Licensing Health Care
    Facilities
425 Fifth Avenue N
Nashville, TN 37247-0530
615-741-7221

TEXAS

Nursing Home Licensure Office
Texas Department of Health
8407 Wall Street
Austin, TX 78756
512-834-6647

UTAH

Division of Occupational and
    Professional Licensing
Heber M. Wells Building
160 East 300 South
P.O. Box 45805
Salt Lake City, UT 84145
801-530-6628

VERMONT

Nursing Home Licensure Office
Department of Health
Licensing and Protection
Ladd Hall
103 South Main Street
Waterbury, VT 05671-2306
802-241-2345

VIRGINIA

Office of Health Facilities
    Regulation
Department of Health
360 Centre, Suite 216
3600 West Broad Street
Richmond, VA 23230
804-367-2102

WASHINGTON

Washinton State Nursing Care
Quality Assurance Commis-
    sion
1300 Southeast Quince Street
P.O. Box 47861
Olympia, WA 98504-7864
206-664-4100

WEST VIRGINIA

Nursing Home Licensure
    Office
Health Facilities and Certifica-
    tion Section
1900 Kanawha Boulevard East
Building 3, Suite 550
Charleston, WV 25305
304-558-0050

WISCONSIN

Bureau of Quality Assurance
Division of Supportive Living
P.O. Box 309
Madison, WI 53701
608-267-7185

WYOMING

Department of Health
Division of Health and Medical
    Services
Medical Facilities
Hathaway Building, Fourth
    Floor
Cheyenne, WY 82002-0717
307-777-7656

Nursing Facility and Alternative Residence Organizations

American Association of Homes and Services for the Aging
901 E Street NW, Suite 500
Washington, DC 20004-2011
202-783-2242
A nonprofit national association of nursing facilities and senior independent living and assisted living residences. It will provide a list of all member facilities in your state, including level of facility, type of sponsorship, number of living units or beds and services offered.

American Health Care Association
12301 L Street, NW
Washington, DC 20005
202-842-4444
A national association of accredited nursing facilities. It will provide a list of its member facilities in your state.

National Citizens' Coalition for Nursing Home Reform
1424 16th Street, NW, #202
Washington, DC 20036-2211
202-332-2275
Monitors enforcement of state and federal laws regarding conditions and practices in nursing facilities and other facilities for the elderly. Although it does not provide referrals to nursing facilities or other residences, it can refer you to local organizations that have information about specific facilities.

Ombudsman Offices

Each state has a central office that can refer you to the long-term care ombudsman who is responsible for any specific nursing facility you are considering or in which you are already residing. Long-term care ombudsmen respond to complaints about long-term care facilities and mediate disputes between residents and the facilities. They are in a unique position to know whether a facility has frequent complaints, and whether the facility responds well to them. There is no charge for their services.

ALABAMA

Commission on Aging
770 Washington Avenue, Suite 470
Montgomery, AL 36130-1851
334-242-5743

ALASKA

Commission on Aging
Box 110209
Juneau, AK 99811
907-465-3250

ARIZONA

Aging and Adult Administration
1717 West Jefferson
Phoenix, AZ 85007
602-542-1233

ARKANSAS

Office on Aging and Adult Services
Department of Human Services
1417 Donaghey, Suite 329
7th and Main Streets
P.O. Box 1437
Little Rock, AR 72203
501-682-8521

CALIFORNIA

California Department on Aging
1600 K Street
Sacramento, CA 95814
916-322-5290

COLORADO

Commission on Aging
1575 Sherman Street
Denver, CO 80203
303-620-4127

CONNECTICUT

Connecticut Department on Aging
25 Sigourney
Hartford, CT 06106
860-424-5370

DELAWARE

Division on Aging
1901 North Dupont Highway
New Castle, DE 19720
302-577-4660

DISTRICT OF COLUMBIA

Office of Aging
441 Fourth Street, NW, Suite 9005
Washington, DC 20001
202-724-5622

FLORIDA

Elder Affairs Department
4040 Esplanade Way
Tallahassee, FL 32399-7000
904-414-2000

GEORGIA

Office of Aging
Department of Human Resources
Two Peachtree Street, NW
Atlanta, GA 30309
404-657-5255

HAWAII

Office on Aging
1 Capitol District
250 South Hotel Street, Suite 107
Honolulu, HI 96813
808-586-0100

IDAHO

Idaho Office on Aging
State House, Room 108
Boise, ID 83720
208-334-3833

ILLINOIS

Department on Aging
421 East Capitol Avenue, Suite
    100
Springfield, IL 62701-1789
217-785-2870

INDIANA

Aging Services Division
402 West Washington
Indianapolis, IN 46207-7083
317-232-1147

IOWA

Department of Elder Affairs
200 10th Street, 3rd Floor
Des Moines, IA 50319
515-281-5187

KANSAS

Department on Aging
915 SW Harrison
Docking State Office Building,
    Room 122 South
Topeka, KS 66612
913-296-4986

KENTUCKY

Division for Aging Services
Department of Human
    Resources
275 East Main Street, 5th Floor
    West
Frankfort, KY 40621
502-564-6930

LOUISIANA

Governor's Office of Elderly
    Affairs
421 North Fourth Street
Baton Rouge, LA 70806
504-342-7100

MAINE

Bureau of Elder and Adult
    Services
State House Station 11
Augusta, ME 04333
207-624-5335

MARYLAND

Maryland Office on Aging
301 West Preston Street, Room
    1007
Baltimore, MD 21201
410-767-1102

MASSACHUSETTS

Massachusetts Executive Office
    of Elder Affairs
One Ashburton Place
Boston, MA 02108
617-727-7550

MICHIGAN

Offices of Services to the Aging
611 West Ottawa Street, 3rd
    Floor
Lansing, MI 48909
517-373-7876

MINNESOTA

Minnesota Board on Aging
444 Lafayette Road
St. Paul, MN 55155-3843
612-296-1531

MISSISSIPPI

Mississippi Council on Aging
750 North State Street
Jackson, MS 39202
601-359-4929

MISSOURI

Division on Aging
Department of Social Services
221 West High Street
Jefferson City, MO 65102
573-751-3082

MONTANA

Senior and Long-Term Care
Department of Public Health &
    Human Services
P.O. Box 4210
Helena, MT 59620
406-444-4209

NEBRASKA

Aging Services
P.O. Box 95026
Lincoln, NE 68509-5026
402-471-4617

NEVADA

Division of Aging Services
Department of Human
    Resources
505 East King Street, Room 600
Carson City, NV 89710
702-486-3545

NEW HAMPSHIRE

Division of Elderly Services
115 Pleasant Street
Concord, NH 03301-3843
603-271-4390

NEW JERSEY

Senior Affairs Division
Department of Health & Senior
    Services
P.O. Box 807
Trenton, NJ 08625-0807
609-292-3766

NEW MEXICO

State Agency on Aging
228 East Palace Avenue
Santa Fe, NM 87501
505-827-7640

NEW YORK

Office for the Aging
Agency Building #2
Empire State Plaza
Albany, NY 12223
518-474-4425

NORTH CAROLINA

North Carolina Department
of Human Resources
Division of Aging
693 Palmer Drive
Raleigh, NC 27603-2001
919-733-3983

NORTH DAKOTA

Aging Services Division
Department of Human Services
600 East Boulevard
Bismarck, ND 58505
701-328-8910

OHIO

Ohio Department on Aging
50 West Broad Street
Columbus, OH 43266-0501
614-466-7246

OKLAHOMA

State Long-Term Care
Ombudsperson
Aging Services
P.O. Box 25352
Oklahoma City, OK 73125
405-521-2327

OREGON

Office of Long-Term Care
Ombudsman
500 Summer Street, NE
Salem, OR 97310
503-945-5811

PENNSYLVANIA

Department of Aging
400 Market Street
Harrisburg, PA 17101-2301
717-783-1550

PUERTO RICO

Gericulture Commission
Department of Social Services
G.P.O. Box 41088
Santurce, PR 00910
787-724-7373

RHODE ISLAND

Rhode Island Department
of Elderly Affairs
160 Pine Street
Providence, RI 02903
401-277-2894

SOUTH CAROLINA

Governor's Division on Aging
202 Arbor Lake Drive, Suite
301
Columbia, SC 29223
803-737-7500

SOUTH DAKOTA

Office of Adult Services and
Aging
Department of Social Services
700 Governor's Drive
Pierre, SD 57501-2291
605-773-3656

TENNESSEE

Commission on Aging
Andrew Jackson Bldg.
500 Deaderick Street, 9th Floor
Nashville, TN 37243-0860
615-741-2056

TEXAS

Texas Department on Aging
P.O. Box 12786 Capitol Station
Austin, TX 78711
512-424-6840

UTAH

Division of Aging and Adult
Services
Department of Social Services
120 North, 200 West, Room
401
Salt Lake City, UT 84103
801-538-3910

VERMONT

Vermont Office on Aging
103 South Main Street
Waterbury, VT 05676
802-241-2400

VIRGINIA

Department for the Aging
1600 Forest Avenue
Richmond, VA 23288
804-662-9333

WASHINGTON

Aging Services
600 Woodland Square Loop SE
P.O. Box 45600
Olympia, WA 98504-5600
360-902-7797

WEST VIRGINIA

Commission on Aging
State Capitol Complex
Charleston, WV 25305
304-348-3317

WISCONSIN

Board on Aging and Long-Term
Care
P.O. 7850
Madison, WI 53707
608-266-3840

WYOMING

Division on Aging
139 Hathoway Building
Cheyenne, WY 82002
307-777-7986

Reverse Mortgage and Home Equity Conversion Assistance

The following organizations can provide information on reverse mortgages and the various other types of home equity conversions that might be available to help finance home care. Remember, though, that these are referrals only, and any individual plan should be examined carefully with a personal financial adviser.

Home Equity
Information Center
601 E Street, NW
Washington, DC 20049
202-434-6030

American Bar Association
Commission on Legal Problems for the Elderly
1800 M Street, NW
Washington, DC 20036
202-662-1000
Ask for the "Attorney's Guide to Home Equity Conversion."

HUD USER
U.S. Department of Housing & Urban Development
P.O. Box 6091
Rockville, MD 20850
301-251-5154
800-245-2691
e-mail: huduser@aspensys.com
Internet: http://www.huduser.aspensys.com84/huduser.html

Viatical Settlement Assistance

The following organizations may give you leads to reputable viatical settlement companies in your area. They may also provide you with some general information about the terms offered in viatical settlement plans. However, they do not answer specific questions about the advisability of entering into a viatical settlement or about the terms of any specific settlement offer. That is still entirely up to you, with the help of an accountant, lawyer or other financial advisor.

Viatical Association of America
800-842-9811

Maintains a list of member companies that must adhere to certain basic standards of financial responsibility.

American Council of Life Insurance
202-624-2000

Your state's Department of Insurance

Look in the "Government Listings" section of the white pages of your telephone book. ■

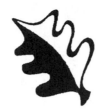

Index

CATALOG

BUSINESS	PRICE	CODE
⊙ The CA Nonprofit Corp Kit (Binder w/CD-ROM)	$39.95	CNP
▣ Consultant & Independent Contractor Agreements (Book w/Disk—PC)	$24.95	CICA
▣ The Corporate Minutes Book (Book w/Disk—PC)	$69.95	CORMI
The Employer's Legal Handbook	$31.95	EMPL
▣ Form Your Own Limited Liability Company (Book w/Disk—PC)	$34.95	LIAB
▣ Hiring Independent Contractors: The Employer's Legal Guide (Book w/Disk—PC)	$29.95	HICI
▣ How to Create a Buy-Sell Agreement and Control the Destiny of your Small Business (Book w/Disk—PC)	$49.95	BSAG
▣ How to Form a California Professional Corporation (Book w/Disk—PC)	$49.95	PROF
▣ How to Form a Nonprofit Corporation (Book w/Disk —PC)—National Edition	$39.95	NNP
⊙ How to Form a Nonprofit Corporation in California	$34.95	NON
▣ How to Form Your Own California Corporation (Binder w/Disk—PC	$39.95	CACI
▣ How to Form Your Own California Corporation (Book w/Disk—PC)	$34.95	CCOR
▣ How to Form Your Own Florida Corporation (Book w/Disk—PC)	$39.95	FLCO
▣ How to Form Your Own New York Corporation (Book w/Disk—PC)	$39.95	NYCO
▣ How to Form Your Own Texas Corporation (Book w/Disk—PC)	$39.95	TCOR
How to Write a Business Plan	$24.95	SBS
The Independent Paralegal's Handbook	$29.95	PARA
Legal Guide for Starting & Running a Small Business, Vol. 1	$24.95	RUNS
▣ Legal Guide for Starting & Running a Small Business, Vol. 2: Legal Forms (Book w/Disk—PC)	$29.95	RUNS2
Marketing Without Advertising	$19.00	MWAD
▣ Music Law (Book w/Disk—PC)	$29.95	ML
Nolo's California Quick Corp (Quick & Legal Series)	$19.95	QINC
⊙ Open Your California Business in 24 Hours (Book w/CD-ROM)	$24.95	OPEN
▣ The Partnership Book: How to Write a Partnership Agreement (Book w/Disk—PC)	$34.95	PART
Sexual Harassment on the Job	$18.95	HARS
Starting & Running a Successful Newsletter or Magazine	$24.95	MAG
Take Charge of Your Workers' Compensation Claim (California Edition)	$29.95	WORK
Tax Savvy for Small Business	$29.95	SAVVY
Trademark: Legal Care for Your Business and Product Name	$34.95	TRD
Wage Slave No More: Law & Taxes for the Self-Employed	$24.95	WAGE
Your Rights in the Workplace	$21.95	YRW

CONSUMER	PRICE	CODE
Fed Up with the Legal System: What's Wrong & How to Fix It	$9.95	LEG
How to Win Your Personal Injury Claim	$26.95	PICL
Nolo's Everyday Law Book	$24.95	EVL
Nolo's Pocket Guide to California Law	$12.95	CLAW
Trouble-Free Travel...And What to Do When Things Go Wrong	$14.95	TRAV

ESTATE PLANNING & PROBATE	PRICE	CODE
8 Ways to Avoid Probate (Quick & Legal Series)	$15.95	PRO8
9 Ways to Avoid Estate Taxes (Quick & Legal Series)	$22.95	ESTX
How to Probate an Estate (California Edition)	$39.95	PAE
Make Your Own Living Trust	$24.95	LITR
Nolo's Law Form Kit: Wills	$14.95	KWL
▣ Nolo's Will Book (Book w/Disk—PC)	$29.95	SWIL

▣ Book with disk
⊙ Book with CD-ROM

CALL 800-992-6656 OR www.nolo.com

	PRICE	CODE
Plan Your Estate	$24.95	NEST
Quick & Legal Will Book (Quick & Legal Series)	$15.95	QUIC

FAMILY MATTERS

	PRICE	CODE
Child Custody: Building Parenting Agreements That Work	$26.95	CUST
The Complete IEP Guide	$24.95	IEP
Divorce & Money: How to Make the Best Financial Decisions During Divorce	$26.95	DIMO
Do Your Own Divorce in Oregon	$19.95	ODIV
Get a Life: You Don't Need a Million to Retire Well	$18.95	LIFE
The Guardianship Book (California Edition)	$39.95	GB
How to Adopt Your Stepchild in California	$34.95	ADOP
How to Raise or Lower Child Support in California (Quick & Legal Series)	$19.95	CHLD
A Legal Guide for Lesbian and Gay Couples	$25.95	LG
The Living Together Kit	$29.95	LTK
Nolo's Pocket Guide to Family Law	$14.95	FLD
Using Divorce Mediation: Save Your Money & Your Sanity	$21.95	UDMD

GOING TO COURT

	PRICE	CODE
Beat Your Ticket: Go To Court and Win! (National Edition)	$19.95	BEYT
Collect Your Court Judgment (California Edition)	$29.95	JUDG
The Criminal Law Handbook: Know Your Rights, Survive the System	$24.95	KYR
Everybody's Guide to Small Claims Court (National Edition)	$18.95	NSCC
Everybody's Guide to Small Claims Court in California	$18.95	CSCC
Fight Your Ticket ... and Win! (California Edition)	$19.95	FYT
How to Change Your Name in California	$34.95	NAME
How to Mediate Your Dispute	$18.95	MEDI
How to Seal Your Juvenile & Criminal Records (California Edition)	$24.95	CRIM
How to Sue For Up to $25,000...and Win!	$29.95	MUNI
Mad at Your Lawyer	$21.95	MAD
Represent Yourself in Court: How to Prepare & Try a Winning Case	$29.95	RYC

HOMEOWNERS, LANDLORDS & TENANTS

		PRICE	CODE
▣	Contractors' and Homeowners' Guide to Mechanics' Liens (Book w/Disk—PC)	$39.95	MIEN
	The Deeds Book (California Edition)	$24.95	DEED
	Dog Law	$14.95	DOG
▣	Every Landlord's Legal Guide (National Edition, Book w/Disk—PC)	$34.95	ELLI
	Every Tenant's Legal Guide	$26.95	EVTEN
	For Sale by Owner in California	$24.95	FSBO
	How to Buy a House in California	$24.95	BHCA
	The Landlord's Law Book, Vol. 1: Rights & Responsibilities (California Edition)	$34.95	LBRT
	The Landlord's Law Book, Vol. 2: Evictions (California Edition)	$34.95	LBEV
	Leases & Rental Agreements (Quick & Legal Series)	$18.95	LEAR
	Neighbor Law: Fences, Trees, Boundaries & Noise	$17.95	NEI
	Renters' Rights (National Edition—Quick & Legal Series))	$15.95	RENT
	Stop Foreclosure Now in California	$29.95	CLOS
	Tenants' Rights (California Edition)	$21.95	CTEN

HUMOR

	PRICE	CODE
29 Reasons Not to Go to Law School	$9.95	29R
Poetic Justice	$9.95	PJ

▣ Book with disk

◉ Book with CD-ROM

		PRICE	CODE

IMMIGRATION

		PRICE	CODE
How to Get a Green Card: Legal Ways to Stay in the U.S.A.		$24.95	GRN
U.S. Immigration Made Easy		$44.95	IMEZ

MONEY MATTERS

		PRICE	CODE
▣ 101 Law Forms for Personal Use (Quick & Legal Series, Book w/disk—PC)		$24.95	SPOT
Bankruptcy: Is It the Right Solution to Your Debt Problems? (Quick & Legal Series)		$15.95	BRS
Chapter 13 Bankruptcy: Repay Your Debts		$29.95	CH13
Credit Repair (Quick & Legal Series)		$15.95	CREP
▣ The Financial Power of Attorney Workbook (Book w/disk—PC)		$24.95	FINPOA
How to File for Chapter 7 Bankruptcy		$26.95	HFB
IRAs, 401(k)s & Other Retirement Plans: Taking Your Money Out		$21.95	RET
Money Troubles: Legal Strategies to Cope With Your Debts		$19.95	MT
Nolo's Law Form Kit: Personal Bankruptcy		$16.95	KBNK
Stand Up to the IRS		$24.95	SIRS
Take Control of Your Student Loans		$19.95	SLOAN

PATENTS AND COPYRIGHTS

		PRICE	CODE
▣ The Copyright Handbook: How to Protect and Use Written Works (Book w/disk—PC)		$29.95	COHA
Copyright Your Software		$24.95	CYS
How to Make Patent Drawings Yourself		$29.95	DRAW
The Inventor's Notebook		$19.95	INOT
▣ License Your Invention (Book w/Disk—PC)		$39.95	LICE
Patent, Copyright & Trademark		$24.95	PCTM
Patent It Yourself		$46.95	PAT
Patent Searching Made Easy		$24.95	PATSE
◉ Software Development: A Legal Guide (Book with CD-ROM)		$44.95	SFT

RESEARCH & REFERENCE

		PRICE	CODE
◉ Government on the Net (Book w/CD-ROM—Windows/Macintosh)		$39.95	GONE
◉ Law on the Net (Book w/CD-ROM Windows/Macintosh)		$39.95	LAWN
Legal Research: How to Find & Understand the Law		$24.95	LRES
Legal Research Made Easy (Video)		$89.95	LRME
◉ Legal Research Online & in the Library (Book w/CD-ROM—Windows/Macintosh)		$39.95	LRO

SENIORS

		PRICE	CODE
Beat the Nursing Home Trap		$21.95	ELD
The Conservatorship Book (California Edition)		$44.95	CNSV
Social Security, Medicare & Pensions		$21.95	SOA

SOFTWARE

Call or check our website at www.nolo.com for special discounts on Software!

		PRICE	CODE
◉ LeaseWriter CD—Windows/Macintosh		$99.95	LWD1
◉ Living Trust Maker CD—Windows/Macintosh		$79.95	LTD2
◉ Small Business Legal Pro 3 CD—Windows/Macintosh		$79.95	SBCD3
◉ Personal RecordKeeper 5.0 CD—Windows/Macintosh		$59.95	RKD5
◉ Patent It Yourself CD—Windows		$229.95	PPC12
◉ WillMaker 7.0 CD—Windows/Macintosh		$69.95	WMD7

Special Upgrade Offer—Get 35% off the latest edition off your Nolo book

It's important to have the most current legal information. Because laws and legal procedures change often, we update our books regularly. To help keep you up-to-date we are extending this special upgrade offer. Cut out and mail the title portion of the cover of your old Nolo book and we'll give you 35% off the retail price of the NEW EDITION of that book when you purchase directly from us. For more information call us at 1-800-992-6656. This offer is to individuals only.

▣ Book with disk

◉ Book with CD-ROM

ORDER FORM

Code	Quantity	Title	Unit price	Total
		Subtotal		
		California residents add Sales Tax		
		Basic Shipping ($3.75)		
		UPS RUSH delivery $8.00–any size order*		
		TOTAL		

Name

Address

(UPS to street address, Priority Mail to P.O. boxes)

* Delivered in 3 business days from receipt of S.F. Bay Area use regular shipping. order.

FOR FASTER SERVICE, USE YOUR CREDIT CARD & OUR TOLL-FREE NUMBERS

Order 24 hours a day   1-800-992-6656
Fax your order   1-800-645-0895
Online   www.nolo.com

METHOD OF PAYMENT

☐ Check enclosed

☐ VISA   ☐ MasterCard   ☐ Discover Card   ☐ American Express

Account #   Expiration Date

Authorizing Signature

Daytime Phone

PRICES SUBJECT TO CHANGE.

VISIT OUR STORE   VISIT US ONLINE

You'll find our complete line of books and software, all at a discount.

BERKELEY
950 Parker Street
Berkeley, CA 94710
1-510-704-2248

on the Internet

www.nolo.com

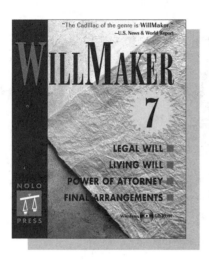
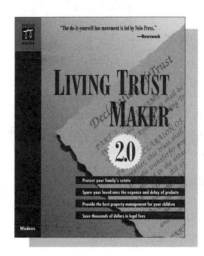

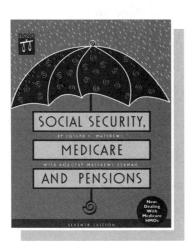
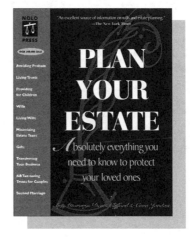

Take 2 minutes & Give us your 2 cents

Your comments make a big difference in the development and revision of Nolo books and software. Please take a few minutes and register your Nolo product—and your comments—with us. Not only will your input make a difference, you'll receive special offers available only to registered owners of Nolo products on our newest books and software. Register now by:

PHONE
1-800-992-6656

FAX
1-800-645-0895

EMAIL
cs@nolo.com

or **MAIL** us
this registration card

REMEMBER:
Little publishers have big ears. We really listen to you.

fold here

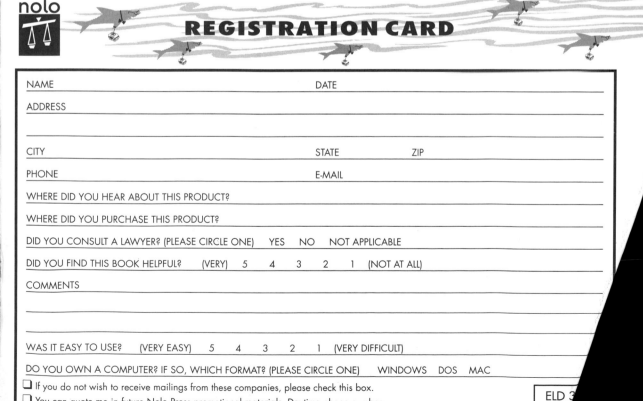

REGISTRATION CARD

nolo

NAME		DATE	
ADDRESS			
CITY		STATE	ZIP
PHONE		E-MAIL	

WHERE DID YOU HEAR ABOUT THIS PRODUCT?

WHERE DID YOU PURCHASE THIS PRODUCT?

DID YOU CONSULT A LAWYER? (PLEASE CIRCLE ONE)   YES   NO   NOT APPLICABLE

DID YOU FIND THIS BOOK HELPFUL?   (VERY)   5   4   3   2   1   (NOT AT ALL)

COMMENTS

WAS IT EASY TO USE?   (VERY EASY)   5   4   3   2   1   (VERY DIFFICULT)

DO YOU OWN A COMPUTER? IF SO, WHICH FORMAT? (PLEASE CIRCLE ONE)   WINDOWS   DOS   MAC

❏ If you do not wish to receive mailings from these companies, please check this box.

❏ You can quote me in future Nolo Press promotional materials. Daytime phone number _____.

ELD 3

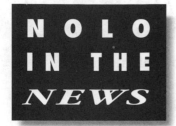
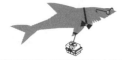

fold here

- -

Place
stamp here

nolo.com
950 Parker Street
Berkeley, CA 94710-9867

ttn: **ELD 3.0**

Take 2 minutes & Give us your 2 cents

Your comments make a big difference in the development and revision of Nolo books and software. Please take a few minutes and register your Nolo product—and your comments—with us. Not only will your input make a difference, you'll receive special offers available only to registered owners of Nolo products on our newest books and software. Register now by:

PHONE
1-800-992-6656

FAX
1-800-645-0895

EMAIL
cs@nolo.com

or **MAIL** us
this registration card

REMEMBER:
Little publishers have big ears. We really listen to you.

fold here

REGISTRATION CARD

NAME _____ DATE _____

ADDRESS _____

_____

CITY _____ STATE _____ ZIP _____

PHONE _____ E-MAIL _____

WHERE DID YOU HEAR ABOUT THIS PRODUCT? _____

WHERE DID YOU PURCHASE THIS PRODUCT? _____

DID YOU CONSULT A LAWYER? (PLEASE CIRCLE ONE)   YES   NO   NOT APPLICABLE

DID YOU FIND THIS BOOK HELPFUL?   (VERY)   5   4   3   2   1   (NOT AT ALL)

COMMENTS _____

_____

_____

WAS IT EASY TO USE?   (VERY EASY)   5   4   3   2   1   (VERY DIFFICULT)

DO YOU OWN A COMPUTER? IF SO, WHICH FORMAT? (PLEASE CIRCLE ONE)   WINDOWS   DOS   MAC

☐ If you do not wish to receive mailings from these companies, please check this box.
☐ You can quote me in future Nolo Press promotional materials. Daytime phone number _____

ELD 3.0

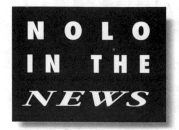

NOLO IN THE NEWS

"Nolo helps lay people perform legal tasks without the aid—or fees—of lawyers."

—USA TODAY

Nolo books are ..."written in plain language, free of legal mumbo jumbo, and spiced with witty personal observations."

—ASSOCIATED PRESS

"...Nolo publications...guide people simply through the how, when, where and why of law."

—WASHINGTON POST

"Increasingly, people who are not lawyers are performing tasks usually regarded as legal work... And consumers, using books like Nolo's, do routine legal work themselves."

—NEW YORK TIMES

"...All of [Nolo's] books are easy-to-understand, are updated regularly, provide pull-out forms...and are often quite moving in their sense of compassion for the struggles of the lay reader."

—SAN FRANCISCO CHRONICLE

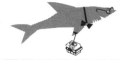

fold here

- -

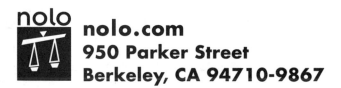

nolo.com
950 Parker Street
Berkeley, CA 94710-9867

Attn: | **ELD 3.0**